chic & slim

TECHNIQUES

10 techniques to make you

chic & slim

à la française

Anne Barone

THE ANNE BARONE COMPANY

Chic & Slim TECHNIQUES:
10 techniques to make you chic & slim *à la française*
Anne Barone

A Chic & Slim Book | Published by The Anne Barone Company
http://www.annebarone.com

Second Edition

Book & Cover Design: Anne Barone
Chic Woman Image: Copyright © iStockphoto / karrapa
Cover Borders: Copyright © Flat-it Type / Ryoichi Tsunekawa
Eiffel Tower Design: Joyce Wells GriggsArt

ISBN Print: 978-1-937066-17-8
ISBN Kindle: 978-1-937066-18-5

Disclaimer Notice to Readers: This book is intended as philosophy and general reference only. It is not a substitute for medical advice or treatment. Every individual's problems with excess weight are unique and complex. You should consult your physician for guidance on any medical condition or health issue and to make certain any products or treatments you use are right and safe for you. The author and publisher disclaim any responsibility for any liability, loss or risk incurred directly or indirectly from the use or application of any of the contents of this publication or from any of the materials, services or products mentioned in the contents of this book or in supplemental materials published on the supporting website *annebarone.com*.

About Author Anne Barone

Once fat and frumpy, in her mid-20s Anne Barone began to learn chic French women's techniques for eating well and staying slim— and for dressing chic on a small budget. She lost 55 pounds and acquired a chic French wardrobe.

Chicer and slimmer, Anne Barone returned to the USA to find a nation growing sloppier and fatter. She decided to share her French secrets.

In 1997, Anne Barone published her first French-inspired book *Chic & Slim: how those chic French women eat all that rich food and still stay slim*. More *Chic & Slim* books followed.

In her books, and on *annebarone.com*, the *Chic & Slim* companion website, Anne Barone continues to share French secrets for dressing chic and staying slim.

Now in her late 60s, she has stayed slim for more than 40 years.

Anne Barone lives in Texas where she is attempting to create a bit of French Provence on the North Texas plains. "Far enough in the country to grow eggplant, apricots and lavender. But close enough to Dallas to make the sales at Neiman Marcus."

more chic & slim by

Anne Barone

chic & slim:
how those chic French women
eat all that rich food
and still stay slim

chic & slim ENCORE:
more about how
French women
dress chic stay slim
—and how you can too!

chic & slim CONNOISSEUR:
using Quality
to be Chic Slim
Safe & Rich

chic & slim TOUJOURS:
aging beutifully
like those
Chic French Women

annebarone.com
chic & slim website

chic & slim
TECHNIQUES

CONTENTS

Bonjour!

Ŧrench women are made, not born.

Parisian-born Véronique Vienne assures us of this fact in her wonderful book *French Style*.

So if French women achieve their chic style, slim figures, serene self-confidence, their femininity and mystique by deliberate effort, then can't any woman acquire that alluring French *je ne sais quoi* if she has a few well-designed techniques to help her?

I believe that any woman, whatever her nationality, wherever she lives, can do just that.

In my previous *Chic & Slim* books, and on the *Chic & Slim* website, *annebarone.com,* I share with you what I have learned over the past decades about how those chic French women achieve their chic style and stay slim. Additionally, you may have read recent media articles about French success at chic and slim. If so, you probably have in mind ways in which you would like to be more like those chic French women.

Surely we would all like to have French women's confidence and serenity. We would like to have a personal style as chic as French women do (on as little money!) and stay as slim while enjoying delicious real food. We would love to maintain the healthy food and lifestyle habits French women do. We would certainly like to maintain their elegant posture. We would love to be as feminine as those *ooh-la-la* French women and enjoy those satisfying relationships with men that make French women's efforts to appear attractive so worthwhile. And we would love to have their aura of mystery, that legendary French mystique that others find so mesmerizing.

No French woman considers herself "finished" before she is 30. Until then, she is a work-in-progress. She is an artist, and she is creating a special work of art: herself. The process she begins as a girl takes years to complete. But years? *Mais non!* We want our changes for success in much less time, don't we?

Designing techniques that will enable you, no matter where you live, to jettison defeating habits and attitudes and replace them with those habits and attitudes you admire in French women *in as little time as possible* is the goal I set for myself when I wrote this book *Chic & Slim Techniques.*

In this updated edition I have added a Special Bonus Resource designed both for those not yet as slim as they wish—as well as for those "effortlessly slim" to help them avoid unforeseen weight gain pitfalls. You will find the two new sections following the techniques.

After one woman read the first two *Chic & Slim* books, she emailed that she was a "long way from being French." Perhaps, with these techniques to speed the process along, you aren't as far as you might think from achieving French chic and slim—and a happy and successful lifestyle.

With these techniques, you may reach your goals in very little time. *Tout de suite!*

So put on your beret (if only in your imagination) set your lips in a seductive French pout, and begin using these techniques to create for yourself a chic style and a slim body *à la française.*

Anne Barone

The Sabrina Technique

THE NEW CHIC & SLIM YOU TECHNIQUE

Sabrina. She was the unattractive, insecure chauffeur's daughter (of the Broadway play and later two Hollywood films) who, with lessons she learned in Paris, returned home changed into a chic, confident, beautiful young woman who captured the millionaire tycoon's heart. But even if we never set foot in France, the French have good lessons for us, just as they had for Sabrina. To learn these useful lessons, you must make a dedicated effort to change. You must be willing to put out some effort to achieve your success.

Positive change requires not just effort, but intelligent effort. Often those efforts are attacked by others who do not wish us to succeed. Sometimes we unconsciously sabotage them ourselves. Deep in our subconscious, many of us have resistance to positive changes that have developed as a result of unfortunate experiences in our lives. How do we insure successful permanent change against the odds that improvements face?

In the 1954 version of *Sabrina*, there is a scene in which Audrey Hepburn as Sabrina is seen sitting at her little desk in her Paris apartment writing her father as she is preparing to return to the USA after finishing her cooking course. She tells her father that in France she has learned more important things than how to prepare French cuisine. "I have learned how to live. How to be in the world, and of the world. And not just to stand aside and watch."

And she declares that she will "never again run away from Life."

If you are overweight, or if you are dressing in a manner that makes you appear less attractive than you really are (or both), could it be that you are running away from Life and hiding beneath your excess flesh and your detracting clothes?

If you are using fat as a protection, what are you afraid of? If there is some trauma in the past, then there may be a valid reason for seeking this security. Some of us need our defenses. But if you are fearful of looking attractive, might not you find other ways of protecting yourself? I understand pepper spray is better than mace. Here in Texas where I live, we have a concealed weapons law and many women carry a gun in their handbag.

To cope with less physical attacks, think of the haughty arrogance those chic French women project. Their attitude says "Approach me if you dare, and do so with respect and politeness." At the time of the death of Princess Margaret of Great Britain in February 2002, an article by Associated Press writer Audrey Woods recalled the Princess's "icy, acid drop stare" with which she could freeze anyone who crossed the line of reserve she set around herself.

Expect people to treat you with politeness and respect (I do) and they will be more likely to respond in that manner (they usually do).

Knowing your destination is one of the basic prerequisites for successful arrival. It's also useful to know precisely where you are when you start out. This next step is so basic that many of you who have read the other *Chic & Slim* books have probably already done it. If not, you should. The step is essential. Even if you have already made your lists, read my cautions.

Keep a note pad around for a day or two and have headings for two lists one for "old" and another for "new." Under "old," write down those defeating habits and attitudes that you want to abandon. Some possibilities are eating quickly, grazing on food while preparing meals, and forgetting to check the backside in the mirror before going out the door (Oh! How it would improve the general aesthetic level of the USA if more people would do this), letting food pushers prompt you to eat food you have no real hunger for, and never taking time for yourself.

Under "new," you might list always sitting for meals, designating some daily boudoir time, regularly pressing clothes, getting to bed before midnight each night, or finding a new hairdresser for a chic haircut.

You can add and subtract from your list as days pass. If you have a computer, creating your lists in a word processing program can be convenient and time saving. And always keep in mind the practicalities. I can outline the most chic, elegant, slim body maintaining, intellectual lifestyle imaginable. The reality is that it is impossible to create and maintain that lifestyle here in a small North Texas city on the time and money that I currently have.

In designing your new lifestyle, remember the good example of the French women's practicality. The French women I have known through the years always seemed to excel at decorating their houses, dressing themselves, preparing meals and organizing entertainment, yet they did not exceed the time and money they had available.

When you do begin to lose weight and improve your appearance, are you prepared for tacky statements from jealous family members and acquaintances? I don't say friends, because surely a "friend" would not make tacky, jealous statements about health improvements. Would they?

When I returned to my home town after my weight loss, some people, who had known me as a fatty, did not immediately recognize me. Others were effusive in their compliments and truly shared my joy that I had lost the fat I had struggled so unsuccessfully to shed as a child and teenager. But not everyone was nice. On that first trip home, I was standing in a downtown store chatting with a family friend when a woman who could always be depended on to insult you walked in. She looked me up and down from head to toe, my former size 18 plus body now fitting nicely in a size 5. "Hello, Anne," she said. "I see your face still breaks out."

Oh dear! I had changed. But she had not.

Will you be able to laugh when you have lost eight of the 25 pounds your doctor has told you to lose, and this tacky coworker goes on for 10 minutes every morning saying how sick you look?

I suggest that in such a case, you tell her you are sick. Tell her you suffer from Barone's Syndrome. The symptoms of this condition are when you have made progress improving your health and some tacky and insecure person says you look sick. Then, mimicking the French actress Juliette Binoche in a scene from the film *The Incredible Lightness of Being,* you begin hopping from one foot to the other and in a gleeful, sing-song chant repeat, "You're jealous! You're jealous! Ha, ha, ha! You're jealous."

Living in less sophisticated societies around the world, I learned the value of ritual in reinforcing change. Coming of age ceremonies in Africa and elsewhere impress upon the mind of the young woman or man that they are no longer children but are ready for the responsibilities and prerogatives of adulthood.

Likewise, we can devise a ritual for impressing on our minds that we are giving up our defeating habits and attitudes and committing ourselves to replacing them with more beneficial habits and attitudes. In a past website article, I recommend the garbage bag technique for getting rid of your guilt about eating foods that were not the best choice for your body. The idea is to write on slips of paper all the unfortunate food practices and incidents about which you feel guilty, put the slips of paper in a garbage bag, tie it up, march out to the dumpster , and throw the bag away. You should then have a sense of liberation from your guilt over this overeating. As I have written elsewhere, I believe that guilt about overeating is often as much responsible for gaining excess weight as the excess calories consumed. You can also use the garbage bag technique to symbolically rid yourself of other defeating habits and attitudes.

Another technique to facilitate change is to take a French name for yourself. (Some of you already have French names so you would have to choose a *different* French name.) Maybe someone named Bobbie Jo who had already eaten a good supper would consume a medium pizza and wash it down with 12 ounces of cola watching three hours of television in the evening. But would someone named Marie-Jeanne or Claire do such a thing? *Non, non, non! Pas possible!*

If you wanted to go to a bit of expense here to reinforce this new thinking about yourself, you might have a medallion made for your key chain engraved with the new name. Or a name plate or calling cards.

Yet another technique I have used when I want to make positive changes for my life is that I write a media profile of the new me. I imagine being interviewed after I have discarded defeating behaviors or inefficient systems. I profile my lifestyle as it is *after* the changes. This profile includes detailed information on my personal style, home decor, my daily routine, my exercise program, the meals I eat and at what time, the china and cutlery I use, the kind of music I listen to, the books I read, my pets, the films I choose, my travel. This profile takes several hours over a period of days to write. It then serves as a guideline for the changes that I attempt to make. It puts the emphasis on the new positive lifestyle rather than on the former lifestyle that is no longer serving me well.

Originally when I began using this technique, I worked in

longhand. Now I use a word processing program on computer. This makes it easy to pull the profile up on screen and read it (at least once a week) for reinforcement. It is also useful to keep a printout in a folder for easy reading in a few spare moments.

Keep your profile in a folder or loose leaf notebook. (Call it your Chic & Slim Lifestyle Notebook.) You can include photos of role models, magazine pages of decor you like, related media articles, anything that gives reinforcement and definition to your goals for yourself. And please, please stick with positive models. No negative images.

If you have no time for writing a profile, talk to yourself as if being interviewed, and then respond. Try this while doing household chores, putting on makeup, or cooking.

Abandon any feelings of resentment that you might have. Life is not fair. Most of us were shortchanged in one department or another. Just about every woman in the world has better legs than mine. Despite staying slim and regular toning exercise, compared to the legs practically every other woman I see wearing shorts or short skirts, mine do not rate very well. The older I get, the further mine seem to be from the norm. Just as I was proofing this technique, I glanced out the window and saw a woman I know is as old as I and who, I am reasonably sure, has never done five minutes leg toning in her whole life. She was wearing short shorts and her legs look really great.

Here is my choice: I can spend time resenting this and agonizing over the cosmic unfairness of it all. Or, I can pull on a pair of jeans that hide the worst of my leg imperfections and get on with my life. If I really want to do something about this, I can spend some money and have some "medical editing."

There are so many things that you can control and change to make your appearance more attractive and your life better.

Concentrate on those. Do not waste time lamenting those things that you cannot change.

I like, have used, and recommend Dr. Nathaniel Branden's self-esteem books and recordings as aids to making positive lifestyle changes. Dr. Branden also has a website *nathanielbranden.com.*

Taking actions consistent with the new chic and slim person we want to be achieves powerful results. Any of us who have successfully let go of defeating habits have likely employed that technique. I still do on a regular basis. At least once a day. I stop myself and say: "What would a chic French woman do in this situation?"

Like so many of us, I have negative tapes playing in my mind telling me that I am not this, or not that, or that I am too this or too that for success in something. And sometimes those negative mind tapes set me on a path to a defeating action. But often I stop myself and think: Is this action or reaction one that is really the person I want to be, or is it the way I was programmed to act or react by the painful experiences in my life? By those painful experiences that made me a fatty and kept me fat for many years. If instead of a fatty growing up in the USA heartland, if I had grown up slim within the French culture and with family members who would have given me good examples and training in how to live successfully as a woman, would I react this way? "What would a chic French woman do?"

The good news is that after repeatedly taking the actions of the person you want to be rather than taking the actions of the person that you were, you begin more and more automatically to take the actions of that person you want to be. You become that new, changed person. Often now I stop and smile to myself realizing that the successful response I have just given to a situation was so-o-o-o French. *Fantastique!*

How You Do It For Chic & Slim Success:

If you are afraid of becoming chic and slim, look for protections other than excess fat and unattractive personal style.

Get a clear idea of the habits and attitudes you wish to discard. Make a list.

Get a clear idea of the habits and attitudes you wish to acquire. Make a list.

Design a ritual to say farewell to the "old you." The garbage bag technique is one possibility. Writing an obituary for the "old you" is another possibility.

Make or purchase a token that you see often that will remind you of the new person you are becoming. Key chain medallion, name plate, business card.

Take daily actions consistent with the chic and slim person you want to be.

Ask yourself: "What would a chic French woman do in this situation?" Then do it.

The Classique Technique

THE MEN-AS-INSPIRATION TECHNIQUE

What is classic? Why is this technique to show you the philosophy behind French women finding men useful motivation to dress chic and stay slim called The *Classique* Technique?

Dictionary definitions for classic include: belonging to the highest rank or class, serving as the established model or standard, having lasting significance or worth, enduring.

A classic holds its value over time; classic design is good and workable. Over time French women have found strong motivation to make the effort to care for themselves and to dress attractively in the attention and positive reaction that men give them for these efforts. And it is not only young French women who receive the rewards for their efforts.

In Dorothy Adelson's *Roughing It On The Rue de la Paix*, her book about her life in Paris, she tells of a party she attended there:

A woman's taste in "arranging herself" was recognized and applauded. Whether she was young or older mattered very little. At one big cocktail party, the two belles were both women in their fifties, *soigneés élégantes*. They had *beaucoup de success*—which, in the French phrase, meant success with the opposite sex. In fact, the value set on experience gave older women the edge.

A further clarification on the *beaucoup de success*. This does not mean that these women "picked up" men at this party. It simply means that men paid attention to these two older women and wanted to talk with them, paid them small courtesies and compliments. These women of a "certain age" were not ignored while the men focused time and attention only on younger women.

I have always wondered which was the cause and which the effect. Did women age 40 and older in France put out effort to be attractive because the French culture is one that admires vintage in women as well as in wine? Or was it that in French culture, older women are appreciated because women over 40 maintain themselves in a manner to evoke appreciation?

One often reads that French men value older French women for their charm and experience. Charm and experience of mature women does not appear to be as greatly valued in the USA. Texas men are known to like their women "green." And we also know it is not only American men in Texas who often demonstrate a preference for young, immature, and inexperienced females.

Yet, for centuries, various French women have been remembered for charming and holding the affections of men decades younger than they. Diane de Poitiers comes to mind. The mistress of Henry II was 20 years older than the king. During the time Henry II was on the throne, Diane de Poitiers reigned as queen of France in all but title.

In *The Book of the Courtesans*, author Susan Griffin tells the story of French writer and courtesan Ninon de Lenclos. She writes that when young Abbe Gedolyn began to pursue Ninon, she put him off. But when she finally agreed to be his lover, she told the young man that he must wait for one month and one day to have her. He agreed. The day came. Susan Griffin writes:

> Happy in her arms at last, he asked her why she had made him wait exactly one month and a day. 'Because today is my birthday,' she answered, 'and I wanted to prove to myself that at the age of seventy, I am still capable of entertaining a lover.'

And just think! Ninon de Lenclos managed to remain capable without cosmetic surgery, hormone replacement therapy, or regular injections of Botox.

Actress Audrey Hepburn's second husband was nine years her junior. After her divorce from the Italian doctor, she found her soul mate and shared the last years of her life with actor Robert Wolders, seven years younger than she.

Even if in France and the rest of Europe, it is easier for a woman to remain desirable when she is in her fifties, sixties, and beyond, there are many, many women in the USA more than 50 who are doing quite nicely in this area, thank you. With more knowledge about nutrition and exercise, and with improvements in medicine, some of us past the half-century mark are more attractive and have more energy than when we were decades younger. I know that I certainly look better and feel better than when I was a severely overweight and acne-plagued teenager.

At the *Chic & Slim* website, I receive wonderful email from women telling me how, though they are in their fifties as I am, that they are having *beaucoup de success* with putting the French-inspired *Chic & Slim* philosophy to work for them. I almost called this technique The Ooh-la-la Technique for reasons, if they are not yet obvious, soon will be. I received an email from a woman who had read the *Chic & Slim* books and was pleased with the results of her efforts toward a chic and elegant personal style. She wrote:

Last week I was waiting for the elevator in the building where I work. I was wearing fitted wool trousers (with high heels, of course), a silk blouse and red lipstick. A co-worker, friend (male) came around the corner and, as God is my witness, stopped cold in his tracks and said, *"Ooh-la-la!"*

Certainly we are pleased when our physician praises our ability to keep our weight in the normal range. (One of the reasons I wrote the original *Chic & Slim* was the encouragement of my doctor who said I should tell others how I did it.) We are cheered when another woman of chic style compliments our appearance. But nothing gives us quite the satisfaction as a compliment or complimenting look from a male. Does not matter whether it be husband, lover, coworker, or a stranger who gives us an appreciative glance as he passes us on the street.

French women find great motivation for looking chic and staying slim in the approving looks, comments, and reactions of men. I can think of no better motivation. Saying *"non, merci"* to piles of greasy pasta, drinking mineral water instead of sugared colas, roasting a chicken instead of bringing home a tub of KFC seems a small price to pay for those heartfelt *ooh-la-las*.

The Paris-born American fashion designer Pauline Trigere, "an elegant symbol of American fashion for more than 50 years," was one of the most vocal advocates of using men for inspiration. In an article titled "Trigere created a design for living as well as for fashion," *Cleveland Plain Dealer* Fashion Editor Evelyn Theiss wrote:

> Fashion designer Pauline Trigere, who always looked about 20 years younger than her age, didn't mind sharing tips on how she achieved that: standing on her head, and having lovers.

Evelyn Theiss's article quotes Cleveland television personality and fitness guru Paige Palmer who knew the designer. She said that Pauline Trigere, "always maintained her posture, her looks and her weight. That's probably why she lived as long as she did." The designer died at age 93 and continued her business, entertaining, and active gardening almost to the end of her life.

Many might not want to take Pauline Trigere's advice too exactly. Instead of standing on our heads, we might achieve that daily reverse of blood flow with a slantboard. (I am an enthusiastic user of a slantboard.) Instead of having lovers, we might find inspiration for our efforts to achieve attractive healthy bodies in the admiring looks and comments of men, including husbands.

A woman described by her interviewer for a *Town & Country* makeup article as "an elegant publishing consultant in Manhattan" said that "being in love is the number one beauty secret—it keeps you incandescent."

But let us give the last word on this topic to Diana Vreeland, who, as editor at *Harper's Bazaar* for 27 years and Editor-in-Chief at *Vogue* for ten years made a career out of advising women on fashion and lifestyle. In *Young At Any Age: thirty-three of the world's most elegant women reveal how they stay beautiful*, Diana Vreeland declares emphatically: "It's impossible for a woman to look really good without a man."

But what if a woman does not have a man in her life, the interviewer asked? To this, Diana Vreeland responded: "If you can't find one, make him up." Invent a man, look really good for him, and a real man will come along, she promises.

How You Do It For Chic & Slim Success:

➤ When tempted to skip a part of your grooming routine and watch a television show instead, picture in your mind a man whose good opinion you value turning away from you to gaze on another woman better groomed.

➤ When tempted to eat food for which your body has no need, picture in your mind the man of your dreams. Ask yourself which you would prefer, at chocolate bar or spending some time with him.

➤ Write a description of the kind of man with whom you would like to have a relationship, find a photo in a magazine or newspaper that shows his style. Then, design a personal style and a lifestyle to please him.

chic & slim Email to Anne

Dear Anne,

I'm a very contented newcomer to your site! Your books, your philosophy, your spirit....have all come into my life at just the perfect time! Just when I'm facing all those transformations that happen around that "certain age", your wealth of new ideas for thinking and living have made me feel as though I'm a teenager again....on the threshold of something very exciting!! In just one week everything about my life seems new and fresh again! I've had an utterly decadent and self indulgent time reading your books and web articles (while sipping tea and taking tiny nibbles of "LU" cookies, of course!) as well as many other materials you've recommended (while sipping tea and taking tiny nibbles of "LU" cookies, of course!).

Every so often I jump up and make some major change in my environment, wardrobe, etc! It's as if I am now looking at everything with new eyes. It is SO GREAT! Oh, and (I almost forgot!)....the morning after! the day I received and devoured your first book I got up and made French Bread from scratch. I used to enjoy doing that years ago when my kids were little...I even grind the wheat fresh. Your recipes are fantastic!

Anyway, who should "coincidentally" show up just as the bread came out but our friend (male) from France! We ended up doing a whole French day with the midday meal lasting all day! He was astounded to see my enthusiasm (and questions for him) for anything French! He has dropped by many more times this week and I've sent him home with baked goodies. He said he's never before seen such enthusiasm for the French since he's been in this country!

Anne, I could go on and on with praise and thanks to you! So many wonderful things are happening as a result of your books. Thank you so very much for your extraordinary efforts. And keep those website articles coming...I so look forward to them and enjoy hearing about what you're doing!

Sincerely,,
Janna in Malibu

The Partout Technique

THE CHIC & SLIM ANYWHERE TECHNIQUE

The email and letters communicate the worry. Women worry that developing a chic personal style *à la française* means they must adopt a body-clinging and stiletto-heeled Parisienne chic. The writers say, "Parisienne chic won't work for my lifestyle where I live."

Most often, they are right.

Smart little suits with body-hugging skirts worn with stiletto heels if you trying to keep up with active toddlers on the playground are not very practical for Mississippi in August. Nor for heading out to work in the morning in Michigan during three weeks of blizzard in January. One thing that Parisienne women have aiding their chic is that the weather never varies greatly in Paris. The extremes of heat and cold found in many regions of the world are rarely a problem in the French capital.

Never fear. French chic is much more than Parisienne chic. French women, depending on where they find themselves, play different variations on the theme of French chic. They can achieve Riviera beach chic or French countryside chic as successfully as Parisienne chic.

Stanley Marcus, long a guiding light of *Neiman Marcus* stores, understood that not only American women in New York had an interest in quality design in fashion. As *Washington Post* Staff

Writer Robin Givhan wrote in a tribute to the legendary retailer at the time of his death in 2002, "Marcus knew that elegance was not tied to geography." He understood this concept so well that back in 1953, Vogue magazine called Dallas's *Neiman Marcus* "Texas with a French accent."

What Stanley Marcus also understood was that women, depending on the region in which they lived, would achieve their chic in different ways. As Robin Givhan explains in the above-mentioned article: "Marcus believed in elegance, equating it with a keen understanding of appropriateness. And in that definition, he tapped into a critical difference between a New York fashion sense and the rest of the country."

Chic must be appropriate to the place in which you live.

In another *Washington Post* fashion article, Lars Nilsson, the new designer for Bill Blass is quoted. "We may do a trunk show in Portland, Oregon, and then in Palm Beach, and people are not going to buy the same things because the climate is so different," he says. "That is the reason that the company has recently developed an all silk flannel in place of the usual wool or cashmere flannel— because people in Palm Beach can wear gray flannel pants and not be too hot."

You can use Paris for inspiration, then design your own appropriate personal style for wherever you live — as did this woman did who recently visited Paris. After she returned to the USA, she emailed:

I visited Paris recently with a friend. Our last evening there, we went to the Opera Garnier and saw a modern ballet. During the intermission we went to the Grand Salon and watched people. I've never seen so many terrific-looking older ladies in my life! It was quite an inspiration to me. Their style was in line with what you mentioned in *Encore* Simple chin-length haircuts. Natural-looking makeup. Very nice pant-suits in neutral colors. Small gold earrings. And that's about it. Of course, they were all very slim. Now, thanks to you, I know how they do it.

No matter where you live, you should be able to purchase a tailored pant suit in a neutral black, gray, brown, or navy, as well as small gold earrings and a decent pair of leather pumps in a color to match your pant suit. Instructions for applying the kind of natural looking makeup French women prefer is there in makeup artist Bobbi Brown's book *Bobbi Brown Beauty*. As for the chic Parisienne hairstyle, I wear a simple chin-length bob. The town to which I drive, where my hairdresser Bev does that haircut, has a population of 2800. A good hairdresser is not defined by geography, but by his or her individual talent and willingness to stay current on styles and cutting techniques.

Wherever French women are, they are always observing other women, looking for good ideas for their own stylish dressing from the informal fashion shows passing by. It is wonderful when, like the woman in the previous email and her friend, you can hang out at the *Opéra Garnier* or a little Parisian sidewalk cafe and watch chic French women. But what about those who do not have time or money to travel to Paris or New York? Where do you get your inspiration for your personal style when so many women you see out and around in the USA are such poor role models for chic?

Fashion magazines, once a wonderful source of inspiration, have, for the most part, become useless as a resource for a good many of us. Unless you are 18-years-old, at least six-feet-one inches tall and are well on your way to anorexia, the photos don't give much idea of what the clothes would actually look like on you. Many fashion photos lately are so arty that you can't really tell how the clothes would look even on the 18-year-old, giraffe-tall anorexics. Prices on the fashions shown are prohibitive for many of us, even for those of us who make quality investment purchases. A lot of us just don't have budgets that allow $2200 casual jackets to wear with $900 *torn* jeans and $1300 handbags.

Television and websites often provide much better opportunities than fashion magazines to see what designs you will find influencing what is for sale. Many television shows are very fashion conscious. Some of the series are watched as much for their fashions as for the plot. (Sometimes the fashions are far better than the plot.) Flicking the remote control almost any time of day will give you a variety of current styles. Also, the women on TV offer models in a wider range of ages and sizes than mostly young, mostly ultra thin, abnormally tall fashion models who are usually camera-angled and PhotoShop re-imaged into even greater perfection than genetic inheritance, their dermatologist, their orthodontist, and their cosmetic surgeon has rendered them.

Even if you don't speak a word of Spanish, tune into the Spanish language stations. You will see some extremely well-dressed women. The thing I particularly like on Spanish language television is these women have thighs. Seeing these attractive women gives hope to those of us, who, even when our weight is in the normal range, find that our genetic and ethnic makeup dictates that we have meat between our knees and hipbone.

On the website *Style.com* you can click on the name of most major designers and see a slide show of what most recently came down their runway, just as if you had attended the shows.

You even get back views in many images. Most designers have websites from which you can order the styles that strike your fancy. And, of course, there are all those catalogs that can be ordered for free or a small price.

If your budget is limited, survey the styles on TV and the Internet and in catalogs for a general idea of what you wish to buy. Then, go to the good stores and examine carefully quality items beyond your budget to see how they are designed and made. Next go to a store (or another department in that store) that is within your budget and see how close you can come to finding that style and quality in an item you can afford.

A fact of life here that French women accept: Shopping for the right chic clothes requires an investment of time and effort. And you must keep a firm grip on fashion magazine editor Diana Vreeland's dictum: Elegance is refusal. You are going to spend a lot more time *not* buying items you find than you are going to spend finding what you require.

FBI operatives could learn things from watching a French woman setting off in search of just the right piece to add to her wardrobe. This is not a fun day out. This is serious business. And if you reach for the same garment on the rack at the same time as a French women in serious shopping mode, if you are smart, you will let her have it. Trust me on this.

With many major ready-to-wear lines offering catalog or website ordering, you need no longer make trips to major cities to find chic style. Though in my mother's generation, a shopping trip to Dallas 125 miles away with a stay in a hotel and lunch in those places that catered to the "ladies who lunch" could be a nice little holiday. My aunt reminisced that on those shopping trips you, of course, wore high-heeled shoes, hat and gloves to shop, especially for *Neiman Marcus*. Today for my "shopping trips," I can sit at my iMac in my nightgown, barefoot, sipping hot tea. I mouse-click my way through the season's collections.

You do you not need to copy Paris or New York for your own personal style. The *Chic & Slim* books are designed to give you the basic underlying principles of French chic. You can then translate those principles to your own lifestyle — as I did for my lifestyle on the Texas Riviera and now North Texas.

I was particularly happy to receive an email some months ago from another Texas woman who related how she was adapting *Chic & Slim* to her own lifestyle.

> When you described your reasons for living where you do, I was a little perplexed as to how I could have a Chic & Slim lifestyle. My husband and I have moved to rural East Texas and are building a log home. The local Wal-Mart and Brookshire's do not have very good produce or bread. I'm not sure about walking on the roads — we are REALLY in the sticks! {sigh} But I thought about it and decided to think like a Frenchwoman living in the countryside. I do know where to get wonderful homemade tortillas and I do go to the city of Tyler some and there is a great French bakery there. When we finish our home I want to put in walking trails—we are on 40 acres so there is plenty of space. Also, I like to cook and plan to learn to make bread. During much of the year there are roadside veggie stands.

As any French woman would, this woman in East Texas is focusing on what she has available, not on what is unavailable. French women take a positive attitude toward their personal style and lifestyle. They don't spend much time on the negatives or on what they can't find or can't afford. They work out clever solutions. They don't look for excuses.

With some wonderful exceptions, however, most of us live in locales where, if we are going to have good bread at reasonable prices, we are going to have to bake it ourselves. Thankfully, you can now buy good bread makers for as little as $60. Using a bread maker, food processor, or mixer with a dough paddle to knead the bread dough takes most of the work out of the process. Fortunately, excellent flours are available in the United States. Many of us will have to drive to another city or order those flours, but the nutritional and taste benefits are worth it, I believe.

Likewise, in many regions of the USA, it takes time to locate what you need for a *Chic & Slim* lifestyle. *Chic & Slim* appeals to a rather exclusive group. What is needed for this lifestyle are not the foods and services most people in the area demand. But if you are persistent, you will find local sources for many quality products.

You will have better success developing a *Chic & Slim* lifestyle no matter where you live if you focus on what is available and how you can use what is available to make your personal style the best possible for you. All it takes is a little French-style daring and confidence in your own ability to make the right style choices for you. I repeat: Right for *you*.

How You Do It For Chic & Slim Success:

➤ In designing your own chic personal style, consider climate and local standards and taboos.

➤ Make a list of the activities for which you must regularly be dressed appropriately and make sure your personal style will be adequate for them.

➤ In the interest of efficient use of time, note what activities you must perform without stopping to change clothes. Make sure your wardrobe includes clothes that can make this transition.

➤ Look for style examples on television and on *style.com*.

➤ Determine what styles look good on you—not someone else.

➤ Check out the expensive shops to see how quality is designed and constructed. If your budget is limited, try to find the closest approximation in lower priced clothes.

Your Personal Style melds your lifestyle, finances, and identity into an overall fashion statement that makes you feel good about yourself and tells the world how to feel about you.... Getting the looks part out of the way allows you to get down to business and the true priorities of your life.

Suzy Gershman
Best Dressed

The process of growth, of being an independent person, of learning who you are and what you want from life, is the real secret of life, happiness, and beauty.... A fulfilled woman is a beautiful woman.

Diane von Furstenberg
Diane von Furstenberg's Book of Beauty

The Mystique Technique

THE AURA OF MYSTERY TECHNIQUE

Mystique. What a delicious French word!

Their mystique, their aura of mystery, ranks as one of the key reasons men find French women so attractive and desirable. But what exactly is mystique? How does having mystique aid French women in developing and maintaining successful and satisfying romantic relationships? How does it aid their relationships with all who know them? More importantly, how can you develop your mystique to enhance your attractiveness and make your relationships more successful and satisfying?

In discussing mystique, it is sometimes easier to describe a woman lacking mystique than to describe one who possesses it.

An example of a woman lacking mystique was an overweight, tightly-permanented woman seated near me on a commuter flight. In the 42 minutes between boarding and landing, she bombarded her seat mate and (most of the rest of the plane since she had a loud, projecting voice) with the story of her life. By the time the plane's wheels touched down on the destination tarmac, we all knew how she met her husband, the problems of her marriage, the saga of her divorce, where she worked, her mother's health, her dog's cute tricks. We were even treated to a brief description of her summer vacation. As we escaped into the airport terminal, there was nothing more any of us wanted to know about that woman. Mystique rating: 0.

Women in the USA in recent decades have not been known for possessing mystique. Though there was a character in a Henry James novel about whom he wrote something to the effect that she was rumored to have shot a man somewhere in Oregon. Not that she had given interviews to CNN and Fox News about the reasons for shooting someone in Oregon, followed immediately by soundbites of interviews with the victim's friends and family. No, it was just that there was some suggestion, quiet whispers . . . no one knew for sure . . . but she might have shot someone, sometime previously, possibly in Oregon. But then it could have been in California. . . . Ah, the mystery. Wouldn't it be interesting if sometime in conversation with her, she might give us hints as to what really happened? That woman had definite mystique.

Women who talk incessantly about themselves squelch any mystique they might have. We know all. Too soon.

A critique of American women's mystique-stifling talk about themselves came in a song by country music star Toby Keith. In his song that hit the top of the Billboard charts in late 2001, Toby Keith complains not just that women talk so incessantly about themselves, but he catalogs the specific topics that he would just as soon not hear about.

As someone who writes about French women, I was interested to find that the specific topics Toby Keith complains about in his song are those that French women would likely not mention in conversation with a man: skin care, wardrobe problems, gynecological topics.

When someone knows the process, the how-it-was-accomplished, the aura of mystery is gone. French women likely would not mention most of the topics on Toby Keith's list because they would see such information as detrimental to their mystique. They do not want too many facts about family, former lovers, work situations to spoil their aura of mystery. They want men to be entranced by the results of their personal style efforts, not discuss the process with them. Besides, French women design their workable personal style and lifestyle to prevent health and wardrobe problems from occurring.

Owen Edwards, writing in an article on makeup in *Town & Country* magazine, said: "I have yet to observe my European wife putting on more than lipstick. I know that something happens in her Continental privacy, but she feels no need to let me see what it is."

And she certainly doesn't talk about it, I will bet.

The French enthusiastically discuss films, books, politics, social problems, the current political scandal. They always seem to have a scandal to discuss. But French men and women seem to have more interesting things to talk about than those mundane matters that inspired Toby Keith's song.

Sometime around the early 1970s, I noticed that many American women began to define being liberated as the right to use profanity and discuss their menstrual problems in mixed company. Sometime around the early 1990s, I noticed many women talking about their problems with menopause. Really, ladies, there are more interesting topics. Especially when people are eating.

In a *Washington Post* article in January 2002, Staff Writer Paul Farhi, writing about Toby Keith's song "I Wanna Talk About Me," quotes radio personality Don Geronimo: "Look, my wife is wonderful. But when I ask her a question, it would be nice if she could condense the answer. All I want is the first and last paragraph, and not all the details in between. That, in essence, is what I pray for in my life."

Women wanting to develop a mystique as entrancing as a French woman's would do well to take Don Geronimo's request as a guideline. The first paragraph and the last, especially on a topic that holds little interest to men. (And don't send me letters and email about equality. We aren't talking about equality here. We are talking about how to have a workable relationship with a man on the French model.)

Two things help your mystique: first spend less time talking, especially on topics for which your listener likely has no interest. Second, become a better listener. This advice applies to conversations with everyone, not just someone with whom you have or want a relationship.

Women would also do well to take a lesson from French women to become better and more sympathetic listeners. Again, and again, I note when someone writes about an interesting and intriguing woman there is a comment or quote about what a good listener she is. Jacqueline Kennedy Onassis, one American woman whose mystique was often noted, was known for focusing completely on a companion in conversation and listening intently. But, you say, so many people are so boring. How can you be expected to give complete attention to a bore who is prattling on about something for which you have no interest?

Again take a lesson from Jackie. She was reported to be adroit at gracefully escaping people who might bore her. One article writer (I have forgotten which) wrote of approaching Jackie and giving his name and saying that (a mutual acquaintance) had suggested he introduce himself to her. 'Oh, and I am so glad you did," Jackie said warmly. And then turned and walked away.

You can always just say "Excuse me," politely, give no other explanation, and walk away. How do they know whether you are rushing to an important business meeting, or desperately needing a bathroom because of medication you are taking? French women's aloofness is also useful when it comes to avoiding bores. Life is short. Spend your listening time on interesting people. Avoid the rest. And have no guilt about not wasting the precious minutes of your life listening to people who talk too much about themselves. If you avoid them, perhaps that will be a good lesson to them that they should find something more interesting to talk about than themselves.

American women are known to complain that men cause problems in a relationship because they are hesitant to express their feelings. From the perspective of my certain age, I think that often when American women complain that American men do not express their feelings, many times they are really complaining that men do not express the feelings for them that these women want men to say they feel. He may not be telling you that he loves you passionately, because he may not. He may just be tolerating you. He may be thinking: This woman keeps nagging me about expressing my feelings, and I'm out of here. You have to earn adoration. And few women have earned adoration complaining about unexpressed feelings.

In any case, women have extraordinary capacity to read the feelings and nonverbal communication of infants and toddlers. Savvy women apply the same techniques to reading the nonverbal communication of men. You may have to read from actions what men cannot say in words. And you may be glad you did. A man's actions may often times be more eloquent than his words. I remember a dinner in which I served a particularly delicious veal scaloppini. I observed one of the male guests eating the dish with much pleasure and gusto. He was a man for whom words did not come easily, but under the inspiration of the moment, he beamed down at his plate and commented, "This stuff is really good. It's not a bit greasy."

If French men are more likely than American men to speak words that thrill a woman, it may be that French women have put much effort into inspiring those feelings. It may be too that the Gallic personality is more inclined than the Anglo-Saxon to expressing passionate feelings in poetic words. And it may be that a Frenchman has had much practice saying the *same* poetic words to a lot of *different* women —sometimes several different women in the same week.

You can always hear more accurately when you listen quietly. French women's serenity that is so often praised is frequently conducted in silence. French women are not chatty for the most part. They can be brilliant conversationalists, but they don't generally chatter. They can sit quietly and contentedly. And many men just want some freedom from verbal input, especially at home. There is value in learning to perfect a quiet tranquility, one in which you are silent, not because you are angry and upset, but silent because you are content.

Given this whole situation of male-female conversation, might it not make sense to choose to have a relationship with someone who talks about things in which you are interested. And might it not also be wise to broaden yourself and take an interest in what your husband and/or lover are interested in?

In a 1986 *Vogue* article, "Anouk Aimee: The Female Mystique," Joan Juliet Buck wrote:

She does not want to give anything away about herself. This doesn't stop her from being friendly, funny, straightforward, touching, full of hope and good sense. . .But ask her a personal question. . .and she looks the other way, giggles, and says, "I hate interviews."

Joan Buck goes on to write; "To spend time with her is to learn a little about the quiet, receptive way to be a woman."

I think the word *receptive* should be noted, particularly in the context of men's willingness or unwillingness to share feelings.

Might it be possible, that if a woman is talking so much about herself, she does not appear to be receptive to information from another? Also I think both men and women are hesitant to share personal feelings with someone who is a "talker." Because you worry that person would share your personal information with too many others.

Town & Country magazine's Special Issue January 2002 "All The Best" featured Catherine Deneuve on the cover. What better poster girl for *the best*? In an article in that issue, film critic Andrew Sarris describes the French actress as "an imperishable icon of all that bespeaks beauty and elegance in French civilization." He quotes from Ephraim Katz's *Film Encyclopedia* entry that described Catherine Deneuve as an "exquisite, fragile beauty, aloof and detached in manner." He says: "I have remained entranced by the mysteries suggested by her marvelously sculpted features, her ever-inquiring eyes, her svelte, often enchantingly attired figure, her modestly revealed charms, which promise so much while exposing so little." He says the actress has retained a core of seriousness that "intoxicates even as it mystifies."

What two better examples of French mystique than these two French actresses Anouk Aimee and Catherine Deneuve, women of a "certain age," yet still alluring and desirable and entrancing men?

The easy thing about developing mystique is that others will do much of the work for you. They will—if you let them. If you don't talk much about yourself, other people will start making things up.

Often, as I related in *Chic & Slim Encore*, other people can make up far more glamorous stories about you than is actual fact. And of course, you neither directly confirm nor deny those stories. That would spoil your mystique.

Developing or perfecting mystique will make you more attractive and desirable—whatever your age.

How You Do It For Chic & Slim Success:

➤ Talk less about yourself.

➤ In casual conversation, avoid sharing personal information more appropriate to conversation with your gynecologist, your hairdresser, your aesthetician, or the clerk at a dress boutique.

➤ Practice listening. Look at the person to whom you are listening. Focus on what they are telling you.

➤ Develop the capacity for quiet tranquility.

➤ To escape bores, say "Excuse me" politely and walk away.

➤ Avoid people who annoy or depress you.

➤ Read or watch at least three media articles a day, read at least one book every few weeks, take an interest in the activities of your community, nation, and world so that you have other topics of conversation besides yourself.

➤ Become knowledgeable on some subject you would be unlikely to know about and bring it up in conversation. If you live in Manhattan, it might be mountain goats. If you live on a farm in Iowa, it might be orchids. People will be intrigued.

Memories of a Chic French Woman

Chic & Slim EMAIL TO ANNE

Hello Anne,

I found your site quite by accident by searching for "making picante sauce" on *Google.com*. I was immediately reminded of a French lady that I worked for during my teen years. I was always amazed at the things that she ate and yet stayed so skinny. She would fix lunch for the both of us and eat as much as I did. Keep in mind that I was a 6'1", 190 pound, high school football player and she was a very petite lady in her late 70's! She would buy the fattest cheeses and bake the most wonderful breads. Then she would make homemade salad dressings and homemade mayonnaise. She would carve roast beef or roast leg-of-lamb and make the best sandwiches I ever had. We would also eat a simple salad and some fresh fruit. I was a teetotaler, but she would drink a little wine with every meal.

She lived alone with two dogs and a parakeet, but she always surrounded herself with beautiful things. She had a lot of art and also painted some herself.

My job was to help her with yard work. She didn't have a yard, but a series of huge flower beds. She also had a small greenhouse and I took care of orchids in it for her.

She would spend (what seemed like) hours every morning pampering herself and then join me in my gardening tasks for an hour or so before going back inside to prepare our meal. Meal preparation took another hour or so even if it was a sandwich. In the evenings, she would paint, entertain friends, or drive to the farmer's market. When any of her friends flew anywhere she would insist they bring her back some fresh fruit. I have eaten fresh bananas that were shaped like baseballs and fresh kiwis that are nothing like the ones you buy in a store.

I never got to eat at a restaurant with her, but she told me that she would never eat out anywhere that did not serve on china plates with silverware. Of course I took that to mean that she never ate fast food.

I think she took a lot of time to enjoy life and the simple pleasures around her. She never got in a hurry about anything. When she was going out to town, she would have me wash her car (a little Mercedes) and warm the engine about 15 minutes before she left.

She lived (and I still live) in the mountains near Asheville, NC. The pace of life here is very slow and people enjoy things (like neighbors) here more than any other place I've been.

I appreciate your web site and reading some of it brings back vivid memories of this lady who enjoyed life.

Patrick in North Carolina

Anne Barone Comments:

Patrick's memories paint a wonderful portrait of a chic French woman. If you have read my other *Chic & Slim* books, recall the factors in French slimness that I described. Observe how this woman's lifestyle shows these factors in practice. She is motivated to devote special attention to her appearance. She takes exercise from her daily activities, in this case gardening. Also note that she has no lawn, just flower beds. Meals she serves are simple, but high quality food is carefully prepared and eaten leisurely and with pleasure. Quality possessions, such as her car, are well cared for.

Best of all, this woman lived her chic French lifestyle in a rural area of the USA. She shows us that you can live chic and slim *à la française* no matter where you reside. Patrick's portrait of this chic French woman provides us with a wonderful role model. *Merci,* Patrick.

The Élégance Technique

THE NO SNACKING TECHNIQUE

In a scene in the 1990 French film *May Fools*, the character played by actress Miou-Miou wanders around the kitchen mindlessly gnawing a carrot stick as she prepares a meal. The third time I saw this movie I realized this carrot chewing was to demonstrate that the character had a problem with food. This between-meal snacking contributed to her excess weight (about 5 pounds as far as I could see, but you know how the French feel about five pounds).

In the USA, eating raw carrot sticks between meals is often a suggested activity for weight reduction. The French consider eating carrot sticks between meals, especially while standing, as contributing to a weight problem.

Americans are the world's champion snackers. And they have the obesity statistics to prove it. Government figures now classify almost than 130 million Americans as either overweight or obese. In their *Washington Post* article, "Supersize Country," Shannon Brownlee, a Markle Senior Fellow at the New America Foundation, and Patti Wolter, a senior editor at *Self* magazine wrote:

> The larger problem lies with the environment. We are surrounded by tasty, cheap, high-fat food, while fruits and vegetables are comparatively more expensive and less readily available. Our suburbs are built without sidewalks, our kids buy candy and soda in the hallways at school, and our sense of portion size is so out of control that we think

a 600-calorie cinnamon bun (about a quarter of the total calories the average man needs per day) is a snack. We could not have designed an environment more conducive to getting fat.

Americans reportedly spend $30 billion a year on snacks. What is interesting to me about this figure is that $30 billion is also the figure I often see given for the amount spent on weight control products in the USA. According to an article by Sandra Gordon, the European Snack Food Association reported that 81 percent of the French surveyed expressed a belief that eating between meals could be a problem or was unhealthy.

Another interesting statistic from Sandra Gordon was that from numerous studies conducted by David Levitsky, professor of nutritional sciences at Cornell, he found that when people snack, they often eat as much at their next meal as if they had not snacked.

I discovered from personal experience that when I snacked between meals, I often wanted *more* food at meals than if I had not snacked. One explanation for this was that I often snacked on highly sugared carbohydrate foods such as cookies. This sugar set off carbohydrate cravings.

I call this technique designed to help you give up snacking The *Elégance* Technique because, for decades, it has been my suspicion that a chief reason French women don't snack between meals is they don't want to run the risk of messing up their lipstick and their clothes. Especially their clothes. Those small wardrobes of quality clothes do not have many spares in case of accident.

This suspicion received support when I read an article by Barbara Bradley, Fashion Editor for the Memphis newspaper *The Commercial Appeal*. The article compared the way women dressed in the USA and Europe. The article quotes Claire Dupuis, manager of apparel fashion marketing for Cotton Incorporated, who notes the confidence European women demonstrate in their style, how they appreciate the details of well constructed clothes, how they pay careful attention to fit, and how they prefer to maintain a wardrobe of a small number of well chosen "investment clothes" to buying many less expensive garments the way American women do.

Barbara Bradley writes: "Okay, but say you're circling the burger palace with fries balanced on your dashboard, and splat! Your $2,000 designer suit suddenly acquires a new Heinz logo. Didn't your investment just tank?"

The response from Claire Dupuis (no mention that she is French, but the name is certainly French) is that most Europeans do not balance fries on their dashboards, nor do they juggle food in their hands as they walk down a street. "They sit down to lunch and eat in a civilized manner," she reminds us.

See what I mean about elegance? You are less likely to smear your mouth or spill food on your clothes if you are eating seated at the table with a napkin in your lap. In situations that permit it, the French are also likely to tie a huge table napkin around their neck to further protect their clothes. Watch those chic French women eat and they practically dive over their plates when they take a bite. Any falling crumbs will tumble directly into the plate. If you want to see a demonstration of this, see the scene in the film *Un Coeur en Hiver (A Heart in Winter)* where the actress Emmanuelle Béart is eating a piece of cheese (The cheese is to revive her, she is claiming to feel weak). She bends her head low over the plate as she takes the tiniest nibble of cheese. While you are watching this, note that this is about as close as you are going to come to a French snack and that the character eats seated with her attention on her cheese. It is clear in the film's context that this nibble of cheese is not something she would do normally, but simply because she is feeling weak and needs some strength-giving fat and protein.

Snacking can also have its perils. As I was writing this book, we had an extreme example of the perils of mindless eating when President George W. Bush, eating a pretzel while watching a sports event on television, reportedly fainted and fell to the floor. Especially for a woman, falling off your chair unconscious with a pretzel in your mouth is not very elegant.

The benefit to giving up snacking is that you will be less likely to do something that will make you appear inelegant. You will be less likely to soil or ruin your chic, well-chosen clothes. You are going to have enough problems keeping the food spills off your lapel when you are concentrating on your food seated at a table.

So how do you make the transition from someone who eats frequently between meals to someone who, as the French do, generally eats only at regular meals or at a seated snack such as afternoon tea? (Remember that I do not consider afternoon tea a snack. Afternoon tea is sanity-saving therapy.)

If you have been snacking between meals, you have your digestive system programmed to respond with the appropriate digestive juices at those times. When you don't eat at that time you have been snacking, at first you will experience discomfort, a "mind hunger"—though, most likely, it will not be true hunger if you have eaten a proper meal.

You will have more success giving up snacks if you do so gradually one snack time at a time. One reason diets don't work is that diets require you to give up all those high calorie snacks you have been stuffing in to gratify every whim of advertising-induced and habit-induced hunger at all hours of the day and night, and substitute something totally unsatisfying. Every morning you have been eating this lovely Danish pastry from this wonderful little bakery with your 10:00 AM *cafe latte*, and now you are supposed to substitute a cheddar rice cake spread with a tablespoon of low fat cottage cheese and a cup of herbal tea. Oh goody, goody! Yuck!

If you are in the habit of eating a bowl of ice cream or <shudder> cereal before bedtime, work on giving up this snack first. Especially the cereal. Remember, cereal is not chic!

If you can delay your dinner until 7:30 or 8:00 PM, as the French do, this will help. Especially when I have eaten my evening meal between 6:00 and 7:00 PM, I find that I often become hungry again if I stay up much beyond 10 PM. So if just-before-bedtime snacking is a problem for you, then you may have to eat your evening meal later, or go to bed a bit earlier. Or both.

When I am getting up around 5:00 AM, I find that I cannot work as productively in that stretch from before dawn until noon unless I eat breakfasts in two shifts. Then when I begin sleeping later, I find that I have to give up that second session of breakfast before it begins to add pounds. If I find myself getting hungry mid-morning, scheduling shopping or other errands during this time makes tolerating the discomfort easier until my body readjusts to the lack of food between breakfast and lunch. If I was sitting at the computer trying to write, the hunger discomfort would distract me and make it difficult for me to concentrate. Usually it only takes three or four days, or at most a week, to get through the worst part of the hunger discomfort. Then, it begins to subside.

If you are thinking of doing an at-home spa weekend, soaking in a luxuriating mineral salt or bubble bath is a good way to get through the snack craving until your digestive system adjusts to no food at this time. Please, please don't tell me you normally snack while soaking in the tub.

A technique that I used for combating a specific snack craving was self-hypnosis tapes. I no longer enjoy real ice cream (too sweet, too cold), but for some reason, several years ago I developed a passion for a specific soft frozen dessert cone sold at Hardee's. There was a Hardee's on the street I always took for shopping, and I reached a point that I could not pass Hardee's any afternoon without stopping for a cone. I found I was thinking up reasons to go shopping so I could stop for a cone. I realized that I must stop the cones before they began to show up on my hips and tummy.

Several years ago subliminal persuasion and self-hypnosis and guided imagery tapes were very popular. You could buy them in any bookstore. Pop one in your cassette tape player, sit or lie down in quiet place where you were unlikely to be disturbed, and listen to the words and music on the tape. Different tapes were designed to help you lose weight, cure insomnia, improve your performance in sports, stop smoking, achieve financial success, and deal with stress.

I cured a decades-old problem with insomnia using a subliminal persuasion/self-hypnosis tape that I bought on a whim in the bookstore one day. Later I happened to find (I think I was sitting in a dentist's waiting room) a magazine how-to article in *Reader's Digest* about scripting your own self-hypnosis tape. I decided to create a tape to help me give up my soft dessert cone snack habit.

Using a weight control self-hypnosis tape whose format I liked as a model, I scripted my own tape to deal with my desert cone obsession and several other habits that I thought it best that I discontinue. I recorded this tape speaking my text into a cassette recorder.

Self-hypnosis tapes are effective when played as you are falling asleep because research has shown that your subconscious can absorb information even when you sleep. It is useful to put the information into your conscious too. I also listened to the tape as I walked for exercise. After about six weeks use, I found myself no longer craving the dessert cones. I haven't tasted one in years. I do think about buying one from time to time when I am somewhere they are sold. But somehow I never do. Something internal invariably stops me.

Of all tapes I have surveyed, I think the best are the guided imagery tapes prepared by psychologist Belleruth Naparstek. Her tapes are sold on her *healthjourneys.com* website. Words and specially composed music make for strong total effectiveness of these tapes. These tapes are rather "new agey" and not for everyone. You can, however, listen to excerpts on the website to help you make a decision if these tapes would be useful to you. The side of the Belleruth tapes with affirmations (positive statements to reinforce positive attitudes and change) may be more acceptable to you.

One problem of eating an extremely low-fat diet is that you often do not feel satisfied in the interval between meals. The French know the value of including healthy fats in the meal to keep you satisfied until the next mealtime and to prevent snacking. That ounce or one-half ounce of high fat cheese to end the meal can help you feel satisfied. On the other hand, ending a meal with a high carbohydrate, high sugar dessert will often have you craving more food not long after you have finished your meal.

If you find that you are snack hungry before bedtime, even after eating a substantial dinner that includes dessert, try substituting a salad and cheese course following the main course of meat and vegetables for the dessert. Eat a salad of fresh lettuces dressed with extra-virgin olive oil and red wine or balsamic vinegar and about one-half to one ounce of an imported cheese or quality American-produced cheese (no Kraft, no Boar's Head, or other industrial cheese food). Skip the high carbohydrate dessert such as cake, pie, cookies, ice cream. Likely you will not want to snack.

Eating a healthy amount of good real food that contains healthy, natural fats and a couple of servings of high fiber vegetables at your meals can prevent the empty feeling that sends you after the chips, candy, and other snacks between meals. Avoiding sugar and too many simple carbohydrates can also sustain your satisfaction.

Much snacking I observe seems to me motivated by greed, that is, a desire for more than one needs, rather than by true hunger. On this topic, philanthropist and writer Brooke Astor wrote in *Vanity Fair* that "To want to enjoy one's dinner is correct, but greed is not. Hunger can be satisfied but greed never can."

And then, greed is not elegant.

Giving up snacking between meals and eating healthy real food seated at meals can help you be as slim and as elegant as chic French women.

How You Do It For Chic & Slim Success:

➤ Give up snacks one snack time at a time.

➤ Use shopping, walking, napping, mineral or bubble baths to distract you from your desire for a snack until your body adjusts to not being fed between meals.

➤ Use prepared or self-scripted self-hypnosis or guided imagery tapes to deal with your snacking problems.

➤ Instead of eating a dessert, end your meal with a salad and cheese course to keep you feeling full and satisfied.

chic & slim Email to Anne

Never before has dieting seemed—dare I say it?—so glamorous and exciting.

Eating well is chic and sexy thanks to your insights!

Cynthia in Yonkers

The Musique Technique

THE MUSIC TECHNIQUE

Are you stressed? Depressed? Do you eat too quickly? Some days, is it simply impossible to find the energy to exercise?

You can use music as an aid to successfully solving a variety of problems that plague you. Music can be a particularly useful aid in helping you eat in a manner that will keep you slim.

The work that details the variety of ways music can heal and help you is Don Campbell's *The Mozart Effect: Tapping the Power of Music to Heal the Body, Strengthen the Mind, and Unlock the Creative Spirit.*

Don Campbell sites the pioneering work of French physician Alfred Tomatis. Dr. Tomatis's research findings established the healing and creative powers of music, particularly the music of Classical composer Wolfgang Amadeus Mozart.

The best known of Dr. Tomatis's treatment successes is the French actor Gerard Depardieu. As an aspiring young actor in the mid-1960s, Gerard Depardieu suffered from such severe stammering he had difficulty speaking. With a few months treatment at Dr. Tomatis's clinic, Gerard Depardieu was on his way to the speaking ease and acting success he enjoys today.

The music used in Gerard Depardieu's treatment was that of Mozart. As Dr. Tomatis explained in his book *Pourquoi Mozart? (Why Mozart?)*, Mozart's music has an extraordinary liberating and healing power. The effect of Mozart's music appears to be stronger and more universally effective than the music of other composers.

As Don Campbell writes:
Clearly, the rhythms, melodies, and high frequencies of Mozart's music stimulate and charge the creative and motivation regions of the brain. But perhaps the key to his greatness is that it all sounds so pure and simple . . . . He is at once deeply mysterious and accessible, and above all without guile. His wit, charm, and simplicity allow us to locate a deeper wisdom in ourselves. To me, Mozart's music is like the great architecture of Moghul India—the Amber Palace in Jaipur, or the Taj Mahal. It is the transparency, the arches, the rhythms within the open space that so profoundly stir the human spirit.

I like Don Campbell's comparison of Mozart's music to jewels of Indo-Islamic architecture. When I lived in India, I became greatly interested in this style of architecture and took advantage of the opportunity to study some of its best known examples located in view of my house. My terrace gave a splendid view of Humayun's Tomb, believed to be the inspiration for the Taj Mahal. Making the pilgrimage to Agra to see the Taj Mahal was one of the unforgettable experiences of my life.

As I keyboard these words into computer memory, I am listening to Mozart's Andante, K 315 played by flutist James Galway with the Chamber Orchestra of Europe. The music is as exquisitely beautiful as the Taj, that concerto in white marble that points its graceful spires into the Indian sky. The music serenades me with a soothing caress that soothes away the distractions and worries and leaves me free to translate my thoughts into words.

Even before I read Don Campbell's book, I had discovered that I did my best writing to the slow movements of music by the Baroque and Classical composers, particularly Vivaldi, Mozart, Handel, Corelli, and Telemann. I also found New Age music good background for working.

In *The Mozart Effect*, Don Campbell writes that "slower Baroque music (Bach, Handel, Vivaldi, Corelli) imparts a sense of stability, order, predictability, and safety and creates a mentally stimulating environment for study or work." Of New Age music he says, "For people living a highly mental, structured life, such music helps them to unwind and float freely."

Not only were they good for creative work, but I found both Baroque and New Age music excellent music to play during meal or teatime to help me relax and enjoy my food. These lovely melodies put me in a frame of mind to remember to "eat elegantly," taking small bites and chewing each bite slowly and carefully.

Stress-producing and unsettling events are unavoidable in everyday life. Particularly as the background music for my sanity-saving afternoon teatime, I find slow, melodic music wonderful help in disconnecting me from problems and troubles and making possible a retreat. In my sanctuary of calm, I can enjoy a cup of tea and an interesting book or article.

Try to imagine a film without background music. In a film, music can define an ambiance that can make us, the viewers, apprehensive, lighthearted, amorous, frightened, or exploding with laughter. Music can intensify our empathized feelings of passion, joy, longing, and patriotism with the characters on the screen. You can put this mood-enhancing facility of music to work for you to help you fight a depression-induced tendency to seek solace in "comfort foods."

If you have defined one of the factors that works against your health and slimness as overeating when you are feeling blue or depressed, try to treat your "down" feelings with a dose of happy music before you treat yourself to everything in the refrigerator you can stuff into your mouth.

Almost all the classic Broadway musicals have spirit-lifting songs. If that guy who says he is going to call doesn't, it may be the time to sing along with "I'm Gonna Wash that Man Right Outa My Hair," from *South Pacific*. I love all the songs from the musical *The Unsinkable Molly Brown*, and "I Ain't Down Yet" is an especially good one to buck you up from a career setback. I was born and raised in Oklahoma and I have had plenty of experience seeing first hand the state's "beautiful mornings" that are so vividly described in the opening number of *Oklahoma!* I remember struggling through a particularly difficult time of my life. Every morning as I prepared my coffee I would sing the musical's opening number, "Oh, What a Beautiful Mornin.'"

The chorus goes: "Oh what a beautiful mornin', oh what a beautiful day. I've got a beautiful feelin' eveything's goin' my way." Everything, of course, did not go my way. But the music gave me a positive attitude that helped me cope with whatever problems and upsets came during the day.

I had already written the above paragraphs when I read *Washington Post* columnist George Will's article about the Broadway revival of *Oklahoma!* George Will points out the play's message is as timely today as we cope with terrorism as it was at the time of its 1943 opening, a dark year in World War II. He quotes historian of Broadway musicals Ethan Mordden who points out that the message in *Oklahoma!* is the unpleasant truth that evil will keep coming at you until you wipe it out. You are going to have to keep coping as best you can with the problems, personal as well as on a global scale. Some good music can keep your spirits up for life's battles.

As careful as I am about nutrition and proper rest for energy, still some days, by the time for my exercise session, I just do not feel as if I possess the energy to walk across the room, much less to put on my walking shoes and go outdoors and walk a couple of miles at a brisk pace—or to make it through an aerobics video.

March music is just that. It is music that has been designed to inspire people to march. Not walk. March. Even when exhausted and battle weary. Move those feet and keep them moving at a brisk pace. Of course the greatest piece of marching music in my opinion is the French national anthem "*La Marseillaise.*" Another great national anthem marching song in the same spirit is the Togolese national anthem. As a United States Peace Corps Volunteer to that West African country, I learned the words and tune to that anthem. It is one of those spirited songs that energizes and raises the pride in the singer.

"The Stars and Stripes Forever," "*Semper Fidelis,*" "The Battle Hymn of the Republic," "Anchors Aweigh," all stir us to pick up our feet and move. If you think you are too tired to exercise, put a march tape in the MP3 or CD player and march in place to the music. Or use march music to set your pace when you are taking a walk outdoors. You will feel like you are leading a parade. Didn't you always want to lead a parade?

Remember that any one type of exercise becomes boring if done every day for years. You need alternatives to your regular exercise to keep exercise pleasurable. Taking your walks or marching in place to march music makes a good alternative exercise. And I have another suggestion. Music, used creatively, can be a powerful aid in helping you cure bad eating habits, lose excess weight, and generally feel more in control of your life.

If listening to Mozart for a couple of months could turn a stammering Frenchman into one of the world's most successful and popular actors, just think what the proper music, used on a regular basis, might do to help you slow your pace of eating and feel serene and competent to deal with your problems. It can also energize you for exercise when you think you would rather just plop on the sofa and stare at the television.

How You Do It For Chic & Slim Success:

➤➤ Use calm soothing music as background to your meals to help you eat more slowly and feel more relaxed at mealtime.

➤➤ Have a collection of happy music to lift your spirits when you feel depressed.

➤➤ Use music to motivate you to exercise.

➤➤ Choose exercise videos with good music. You will enjoy your workouts more and be more likely to use these tapes.

➤➤ Avoid restaurants that use loud, jazzy music to make you eat more food quickly.

Music Resources:

Looking through your own music collection, you likely will find music that you can put to use in your *Chic & Slim* efforts. Following is a list of some of the albums in my own music collection that I use for just the purposes described in this technique. Most of these albums are available in both CD and MP3 formats. For some, *Amazon.com* currently offers the MP3 version free with the purchase of the CD version. Most of the albums are available from the iTunes store as well as *Amazon.com* and other music vendors.

Mozart Adagios Decca (2 CD set) – Time 145:57
Probably the best "slow Mozart" value for the money. The cover blurb says: "Mozart's slow movements contain some of the most beautiful and peaceful melodies ever written."

Mozart for Relaxation RCA Victor – Time 68:01
Familiar Mozart selections exquisitely played.

Mozart's Music for the Night with Sounds of the River Eclipse Music Corp
Time: 64:22 Sounds of Mozart blended with sounds of a flowing river.

Vivaldi Adagios Decca (2 CD set) – Time: 2 hours+ Soothing and peaceful. Vivaldi's adagios are as beautiful and tranquil as Mozart's.

Adagio: Music for Silent Moments Arte Nova – Time: 78:52
Lovely adagios from Bach, Schubert, Elgar, Holst, and Larsson.

Music for Meditation Vol. 1 Creative Music – Time: 56:31
Peaceful classical music at an economical price.

Largo NAXOS - Time: 74:45
Slow, tranquil movements by Baroque composers. Lovely.

25 Baroque Favorites Vox Cameo Classics – Time: 70+ Min.
Beautiful relaxing, elegant music from the Baroque era.

The Jane Austen Companion Nimbus Records - Time: 1:10:45
Particularly the Boyce symphonies provide formality with lively spirit found in Jane Austen's characters. Perfect background music for reading Jane Austen and sipping a cup of afternoon tea.

Italian Harp Music Naxos – Time:1:05:38
Claudia Antonelli's selections of Italian Baroque, Classical and Romantic harp music. Soothing and rejuvenating when tired and stressed.

Telemann Oboe Concertos, Vol 1 Regis Records – Time 1:08:00
Telemann's oboe concertos have a charm and energy that lifts spirits.

Dowland: Lachrimae Hyperion Records Limited – Time: 1:09:00
The cream of Elizabethan lute music of the English Renaissance by a master composer. For your thoughtful moments.

Beyond the Horizon Real Music – Time: 35 min. Hilary Stagg's electronically amplified Irish folk harp. Soothing New Age music with a crystal elegance.

Peace of Mind: *Relaxation* Compose Records – Time: 59:12
Peaceful and relaxing New Age piano music. Calming and restoring.

Highland Cathedral Scotdisc – Time: 1:06:58
The Royal Scots Dragoon Guards' bagpipes will set your feet marching.

chic & slim Email to Anne

Dear Anne,

Thank you very much for sending out my order of your two books so quickly. I wasn't quite sure what to expect from your books. However your books (along with some of my own research) have already made a major difference in my life and my family's life in just one week.

I have stopped dieting or counting calories. I shop now for "real" food. My husband and I sit down at the table for more leisurely family breakfasts and dinners now. We have a small half glass of red wine with dinner instead of soda pop.

In one week:

I have lost 3 pounds.

My husband seems happier and less stressed.

I feel closer to my husband since we talk at breakfast and dinnertime.

I'm sleeping better and my sleep problems seem to be gone.

I have more energy and time to play with my active baby daughter.

All this and more without one bit of dieting!

I am looking forward to implementing more of your commonsense, helpful tips in the future. You don't know how thankful I am that I found your books by accident during a web search. Please ignore your critics and keep up the good work. I feel it is only a matter of time before your books will become word-of-mouth bestsellers.

Best Wishes,
Paula in New York

La Résistance Technique

THE SUGAR REDUCTION TECHNIQUE

During the occupation of France during World War II, an organization that came to be known as *la Résistance* fought the invader. In the last several decades, refined sugar has invaded many foods Americans eat. Like those brave French men and women of *la Résistance* who fought the invader during that second world war, in order to live the *Chic & Slim* lifestyle, we must make an effort to fight off the invasion of refined sugar into our diet.

If you want to make only one modification in your eating for achieving and maintaining a normal weight and improvement in your general health, reducing a regular high consumption of refined sugar and processed carbohydrates is the one to make.

Reading the labels of many foods sold as a low-fat version of that food, you find that they have substituted various forms of sugar: corn syrup, dextrose, lactose, maltose, sucrose, fructose or plain old granulated sugar for the fat in the regular version. "Low-fat" cream cheese is one example that comes to mind. In *Chic & Slim Encore*, the second of my *Chic & Slim* books, I analyze a faux fish product prominently labeled "low-fat" that used about five kinds of sugar. By the way, the stuff tasted like fish poached in children's cough syrup.

What's wrong with eating lots of refined sugar?

In the bestseller *Sugar Busters! : Cut Sugar to Trim Fat*, the authors explain that sugar stimulates the pancreas to secrete insulin. Insulin is needed by our bodies for regulating our blood sugar level, but when our bodies overproduce insulin, we get undesired results. Excess sugar is stored in our bodies as fat. Burning of already stored fat is inhibited. Our livers start making cholesterol that we certainly don't need.

If we eat too much refined sugar, the problems are: (a) we can't burn the fat we already have, (b) we gain even more fat, and (c) cholesterol builds up in our arteries. (Sounds like what has been happening to the health of a lot of people in the USA in the past several decades, doesn't it?)

Eating too much sugar can make us not only overweight, but overweight with heart problems. Oh dear!

Recently research points to a frightening connection between sugar consumption and cancer. For a full explanation you can read the first nine chapters of *Sugar Busters!* And this is probably the place to say that I applaud the book's authors for creating a book that has brought the problem of excessive sugar consumption to the attention of millions of people in the USA. We have a serious, serious problem here. Another, more recent book with an excellent though technical explanation of dangers of excess sugar consumption is *Fat Chance: Beating the Odds Against Sugar, Processed Food, Obesity, and Disease* by Dr. Robert H. Lustig. In both books the authors offer a detailed solution to this problem. I know from personal experience, however, that it is possible to follow programs less extreme as these books recommend and still stay slim using my French-inspired *Chic & Slim* system.

The *Sugar Busters!* program prohibits potatoes, white bread, beets, and carrots (among other foods). As for potatoes, the French eat about three times as many as Americans. They eat carrots and beets prepared in a variety of ways. (In any case, I really don't think overconsumption of beets and carrots rates at the top of the list of factors in obesity in the USA.) And those wonderful baguettes the French eat are certainly made with white flour, though it is a quality, unbleached white flour. Additionally French bread does not contain sugar and chemicals as much bread consumed in the USA does.

Another point in *Sugar Busters!* with which I am not in complete agreement is their lack of restriction on beverages and foods sweetened with aspartame. The product is sold under a variety of product names and labels. The book's only statement on aspartame that I could find said (in small print on page 126 of my copy of *SugarBusters!*): "Artificial sweeteners are not harmful to the vast majority of individuals. However, they have no nutritional value."

Puritanism in the USA wants people to suffer to lose weight, so when I read articles against the use of some particular diet aid, I always try to evaluate if there really are dangers that have been proven by unbiased scientific testing, or whether the negative media is only Puritanism at work.

But I never felt entirely comfortable with even with limited aspartame use. A number of my friends who have extensive knowledge of chemistry and medicine avoid aspartame as if it were anthrax. (That should have told me something.) In connection with writing this section of the book, I researched the scenario that resulted in the FDA approval of aspartame. What my research uncovered makes me sufficiently uneasy about the approval process for that product that I am very thankful I was cautious in my aspartame use. At this time, I am no longer using aspartame.

The French believe that in the long run, using artificial sweeteners will make you eat more sugar instead of less because you will want sweet foods sweeter. Many sweet French foods just aren't as sweet as similar foods in the USA. For instance, the flan I was served in French homes was invariably much less sweet than pudding I ate in American homes.

When I began to observe the French, the most dramatic difference I noticed in the way the French ate and the way that I had always eaten as a fatty was the amount of refined sugar consumed both in foods and in beverages. I was, after all, part of the "Pepsi generation,"and I shudder to remember how many sugared cola soft drinks I consumed as a fatty. Not to mention all that fruit punch served at all those receptions and parties. In our family, there was ample jam or jelly (usually homemade) spread on breakfast toast. Cake, pie, or cookies and ice cream were served after every lunch and dinner. I observed that when the French ate desserts (and often they didn't), they ate these dinky little servings. Accustomed to large American dessert servings, I found the French-sized servings of desserts disappointingly small.

Another thing I observed about French desserts was that there was generally protein in the dessert in the form of milk or egg white or nuts. When they drank sugar-sweetened beverages, the French sipped a few fluid ounces slowly. A small glass of beverage would be sipped for hours.

If you live in the USA and you eat much food prepared outside your home, or if you use many prepared or convenience foods, you will have difficulty keeping your sugar consumption as low as the French do. Many commercial foods contain sugar in one form or another. You often see "modified food starch" listed in the ingredients. In *SugarBusters!* the authors say that starch is simply a large sugar molecule. In our digestive tracts starch quickly becomes glucose. According to that explanation, eating modified food starch seems to produce the same results as eating sugar. It is difficult these days to find a brand of cottage cheese that does not contain modified food starch. A shame, I think, to add an unhealthy ingredient to a cheese that has long been a healthy form of dairy.

Read the labels. Know what you are eating. But a warning: it can be scary knowing what processed foods actually contain. And if you want to be really, really terrified about sugar and processed foods, read *Fat Chance: Beating the Odds Against Sugar, Processed*

Food, Obesity, and Disease. This book by Robert H. Lustig, M.D. published in 2012 has the benefit of a decade and a half more medical research than *Sugar Busters!* published in 1998. Not only does Dr. Lustig define the complexity of problems of the current American diet and their relationship to the obesity epidemic and disease, he also prescribes specific and practical solutions for both individual eating and government policy.

In *Fat Chance*, Dr. Lustig "documents the science and politics that have led to personal misery and public crisis—the pandemic of obesity and chronic disease."

If you regularly drink sugared soft drinks, lemonades, fruit juices with added sugar, fruit punches, most beers, sweet white wines, the most dramatic reduction in calories from sugar in your diet would be to give up those sugared beverages. Sugar is added in the fermentation process to American wines, I am told. Perhaps that is why I find American wine more intoxicating that a good French wine. The French prefer dry (less sweet) red wines. Americans like sweeter wines, particularly sweet white wines. If you drink wine, you will usually consume less sugar if you drink a dry red wine as the French do rather than a sweet white such as a Zinfandel. In any case, American Zinfandels always taste to me like fermented 7-Up.

One of the first French-inspired modifications I made to my lifestyle was substituting a glass of mineral water with a squeeze of lemon or lime for carbonated cola drinks I had been drinking most of my fatty life. The naturally carbonated mineral waters such as Perrier (French), Apollinaris (German) or San Pellegrino (Italian) make good substitutes for carbonated soft drinks. All these have natural carbonation. If you try to go directly to a nongaseous mineral water such as Evian, it may taste too flat to satisfy. And be warned. Not all bottled waters are mineral waters.

So many bottled waters you find on your supermarket shelf

are just filtered tap water put in bottles. Look for the source (you hope it is high in some unpolluted mountains somewhere) and a listing of the mineral content on the label. (Unfortunately not many American mineral waters have these. They just list an 800 number or website where they will answer questions.) If the bottle label says something like filtered tap water from the water supply of some American city, that is *not* mineral water. You might as well just buy yourself a Brita or a Bodum pitcher and filter your own tap water. It will be a lot cheaper. And you won't be cluttering up the landfill with all those plastic bottles.

Another good substitute for sugared beverages is to drink herbal tea chilled or over ice. I drink herbal teas unsweetened. But even if you add a teaspoon of honey, molasses or sugar to sweeten a glass or cup of the tea, you will be cutting back considerably from the sugar contained in a carbonated cola beverage. Most carbonated soft drinks contain about nine teaspoons of sugar in each 12-ounce can of beverage.

Peppermint tea can be wonderfully refreshing in hot weather, as can lemongrass herbal tea. Another herbal favorite is lemon verbena, a good choice for afternoon tea for those who avoid caffeine. A friend's favorite hot weather beverage is green tea with peach served over ice. An elegant beverage for a summer afternoon.

Cutting back on cookies, cakes, pies, doughnuts, sweet rolls, ice cream, and candy is such an obvious way to cut your sugar consumption that I feel almost silly mentioning it. But when you cut down on the cookies, cakes, pies, doughnuts, sweet rolls, ice cream, and candy, what are you going to eat in their place? They are obviously important to you, or you would not be eating them.

If you have been eating a lot of sugared foods, you are going to have to cut back gradually if you want that reduction to be a permanent change in your diet. If you have read the other *Chic &*

Slim books and the postings on the *Chic & Slim* website, you may be weary of me using the word gradually. The reason I keep saying gradually is that is the way our bodies allow us to make changes that become permanent without too much discomfort. If you try to make big changes quickly, your mind and body will fight you. And your mind and body will probably win. You will go back to your well-established, defeating food habits.

On the topic of change made gradually, I offer you this example. Thane Peterson, *Business Week Online* Contributing Editor, made the following observation in one of his weekly Moveable Feast columns, titled "Why So Few French Are Fat." He writes about how Ruth Reichl, editor-in-chief of *Gourmet* magazine, described in a column "how she had always been a bit overweight until one day she decided to eat exactly what she wanted. Miraculously, she gradually lost 30 pounds." Note the word "gradually."

Thane Peterson comments: "As the French have known for years, if what you want to eat is good, fresh food in the company of others, keeping your weight down isn't all that hard for most people."

Please note that he said "...if what you want to eat is *good, fresh food*..." This is important. If what you want to eat is humongous quantities of nutritionless *junque* food and fast food that includes no fresh fruit and no low-calorie green vegetables, and a lot of carbohydrates made from refined white flour, then it will certainly take a miracle for you to lose weight and remain slim permanently.

If you eat commercially-made jam on your breakfast bread, you are eating mostly sugar. Today most American brands of factory-made jams and jellies are just corn syrup and sugar with little fruit. You can buy brands of all fruit jams or jellies, though I believe by law they have to be labeled "spreads" or some such thing. These all-fruit jams are generally more expensive than the corn syrup and sugar jams, jellies, and preserves because it is much less expensive to put corn syrup, food color and pectin in a jar than fruit. Also you do not have to wash, peel, seed, and chop corn syrup, food color, and pectin.

In the typical French kitchen, you find jars of homemade jams and preserves lined up on a shelf. The French make these *confitures* from fresh or dried fruit and sweeten them with grape or apple juice to make an all-fruit recipe. I have recipes for a quick microwave version of this jam in the original *Chic & Slim* as well as *Chic & Slim Encore*. If you don't use a microwave, you can prepare the jam on top of the stove using traditional jam-making techniques included in any standard cookbook.

For breakfast I often eat a wedge of my Barone Breakfast Bread. This bread is made without sugar of any kind and is based on Irish soda bread. Eating too much of products made with wheat has been shown to interfere with metabolism; so I have been making my bread using a combination of other flours: whole grain rye, whole grain soy, spelt, buckwheat, corn, old fashioned rolled oats, and ground flax seed. I always bake this bread in my old-faithful cast-iron skillet. This recipe makes a heavy, stick-to-your-ribs bread that I spread with butter or a nut butter. Almond or walnut can be heavenly. For a while, I even became rather fond of sunflower seed butter, though I never thought of it as heavenly. Just a sort of nutty taste. Sunflower seed butter is usually cheaper than almond or walnut butter. I eat it when feeling frugal.

Note: As I update this book, I must mention that in the past several years, I have found it almost impossible to find the quality of nut butters that I was enjoying at the time I originally wrote this book. Even those that list no added ingredients on the label seem to be much oilier than in the past. Now I often anoint the bread with organic flaxseed oil, a great source of omega-3s and giving a nutty taste when combined with the bread. Though I admit that flaxseed oil by itself does not appeal to my taste buds.

Sometimes on my breakfast bread or muffin, I use a basic white goat cheese or a Mexican cheese, *queso fresco* and top this with one of my homemade all-fruit jams. When I visited my son, his neighborhood supermarket sold a nice Danish feta that was good breakfast eating spread on whole wheat sourdough.

Ricotta cheese is also good for spreading on your breakfast bread. As is cream cheese. Sometimes I eat yogurt cheese on Barone Breakfast Bread or other morning breads. Yogurt cheese is easy to make from plain yogurt if you have a tea strainer lined with a couple of coffee filters.

For afternoon tea, I make a variety of sugarless pastries. Oatmeal and other muffins baked without sugar can be given sweetness by sprinkling on a bit of sweetener at the time of serving, or by spreading with a little all-fruit jam. I also make a sugarless cheesecake, a wedge of which can be topped with ricotta or yogurt and fresh fruit.

More and more, however, I am finding that I enjoy a sandwich rather than a sweet pastry with afternoon tea. Curried chicken salad, egg salad, tomato and cheese, or the traditional cucumber sandwich for tea are favorites. All these sandwiches are delicious made with rye or whole grain bread. These fillings also work well on gluten-free crackers.

Since I rarely eat dessert at the end of a meal, this sometimes creates a potential problem when I am eating a meal in someone else's home. If the hostess or host has gone to the effort to create or purchase a spectacular dessert, she (or he) may be unhappy when I refuse what has taken so much time and effort to create — or money to purchase. I will often ask my hostess or host if I may take my serving home with me.

Of course, these party desserts are invariably made with much sugar. I can reduce the amount of sugar I consume in my afternoon tea pastry by scraping off the frosting (from cakes) and then topping a half or third of the serving with cheese or fresh fruit. If the dessert is pie, I only eat half or third of the serving and top that with cheese and fresh fruit. If it is a fruit pie, I will sometimes add only cheese. A good sharp Wisconsin cheddar, or its English cousin Cheshire, is wonderful on apple or pear pie. Cheshire is an old cheese (it has been around since the 12th century) and a bit firmer and crumblier than cheddar. Lovely with fruit. Feta (one that is not too salty) is good crumbled on peach or berry pie. Valbreso feta, a French sheep's milk cheese works well.

Though I often blame advertising for causing Americans to overeat foods they would best avoid, one positive change in American eating habits resulted from food advertising. Those clever advertisements for Pace Picante Sauce (The weathered Texas cowboys tasting the inferior sauce and saying with a grimace, "This stuff was made in New York City!") weaned many Americans away from highly sugared ketchup, replacing it with an unsugared condiment that contained vegetables. In fact, according to an *austinchronicle.com* posting, by 1992, salsa had replaced ketchup as America's number one condiment.

Thank you, Pace of San Antonio.

The good news is that if you make an effort to cut back on the refined sugar in your diet, your body will help you. I eat so little refined sugar now that when I do eat an American size serving of pie or cake, I feel so ill afterward that the memory of how miserable I was stops me when I am again tempted to so injudiciously indulge.

One more morsel of "Anne Barone's voice of experience" advice. The amount of refined sugar in my diet is now very low. But sometimes I find that I am eating more sugared foods. (This can happen during the Thanksgiving to New Year's holiday season.) I look in my cupboard and see a package of cookies there that I have occasionally eaten as my pastry with my afternoon tea when I had nothing better available. Only three cookies left, I observe. So this idea pops into my head that I will just eat those cookies and get rid of them. Banish temptation in one quick effort.

Do I need to tell you that this eat-it-up-to-get-rid-of-it is a *very bad* idea? If you are tempted to eat a large quantity of sugared foods in an effort to rid the pantry of them, don't. Throw those cookies or cupcakes or whatever in the garbage. Be sure it is the yucky part of the garbage from which you will not retrieve them.

Eating up the supply of cookies or cake or whatever that is left so you can start a virtuous, sugar-free tomorrow is a very bad idea. Anne Barone's voice of experience speaks.

How You Do It For Chic & Slim Success:

➤ Identify foods and beverages that are adding large amounts of sugar to your daily food intake.

➤ Gradually eliminate the major sources of sugar in your diet.

➤ Look to all-fruit jams and to breads and muffins made without sugar to replace the bread and jam you have been eating.

➤ Read *Fat Chance: Beating the Odds Against Sugar, Processed Food, Obesity, and Disease* by Robert H. Lustig to fully understand the dangers of sugars and processed foods and how you can eliminate them for better health and appearance.

➤ Let your body be your ally in eliminating sugar from your diet.

➤ Like French women, instead of carbonated soft drinks, have a glass of mineral water with a squeeze of lemon or lime, or drink a chilled herbal tea.

➤ End your meals with about one-half to one ounce of high fat cheese rather than a highly-sugared dessert.

And then there is Stevia . . .

Without stevia, I could not stay slim.

No, that statement is too strong. More accurately: Without stevia, I could not stay slim—yet still enjoy the quantity and quality of sweet pastries, jams and beverages that I do.

Stevia makes staying slim sweeter.

Using stevia also makes it easier for me to avoid health problems associated with too much sugar in the diet. For one reason or another I find all other replacements for sugar unsatisfactory.

At the time I wrote the original version of this book, I had only begun to use stevia to replace granulated sugar in sweetened foods and beverages. Now, as I write this updated version of *Techniques*, I have used stevia for more than 10 years. Stevia has replaced cane sugar in my food preparation.

Do I ever eat foods containing cane sugar? Certainly. But I keep my consumption of those foods infrequent. A commercial cookie now and then. Dessert at dinner at someone's home or other special dinner. But if the label lists high fructose corn syrup (or any of the aliases the food industry has created to camouflage the presence of high fructose corn syrup) I avoid that food.

Given my decade's experience with stevia, I believe that I can claim a certain expertise on the sweetener. In this section, I will share with you what I have learned that might be helpful to you.

What Exactly Is Stevia?

Stevia is a natural plant product used for centuries in South America—and, for the past 40 years, in Japan—to replace sugar for sweetness in various dishes. Neither the South Americans nor the Japanese seem to have suffered any problems related to this long-term use.

Botanical name for this plant native to Paraguay is *Stevia rebaudiana*. It is the sweetest known natural substance. Stevia leaves are 10 to 15 times as sweet as table sugar. Extracts from stevia leaves range from 100 to 300 times as sweet. Stevia has virtually no calories, doesn't raise blood-sugar levels, nor promotes tooth decay. Stevia is considered safe for most diabetics. While artificial sweeteners have a chemical aftertaste, when stevia's aftertaste is detectable, it is a more natural licorice flavor. Happily the extraction and preparation processes of stevia have been improving. Many stevias currently on the market have little aftertaste when used in food or beverages.

Many Brands Of Stevia Are Unsatisfactory To Me

In the first draft of this update, for the heading I wrote: Many Brands of Stevia Are Terrible. There I was, indulging again in inaccurate hyperbole. But "unsatisfactory to me" is both fair and accurate—yet requiring further clarification.

Many brands of stevia I have tried over the years were unsatisfactory for one or more of four principal reasons.

The first, and most important, reason I found a stevia unsatisfactory is sweetening ability. Some brands I tried just did not provide much noticeable sweetness to the foods or beverages to which I added them. Second, many brands of stevia I find on the shelves of my local supermarkets are overpriced. Other brands deliver an equal or better product at a lower price. Third, a number of versions of stevia have added ingredients I find unacceptable for one reason or another. The fourth reason no doubt equals the first in importance. Stevia's sweet is different from sugar's sweet. Many people taste stevia and simply do not like stevia's sweet. It is too different from the sugar taste they have become accustomed to over their lifetime. I understand. I did not much like stevia's sweet either when I first tried the product. But there are definitely ways to overcome that problem. I begin to explain in the next section.

So, if you tried stevia in the past and decided it was not for you, read the rest I have to say about stevia. You might decide to give stevia another chance. (And save yourself a lot of calories and other negative effects of sugar.)

Actually, I find so many brands of stevia unsatisfactory that I must order my preferred brand of stevia online because I cannot find it for sale locally, even though my supermarkets offer a half dozen brands. Later in this section I will tell you about those brands that I find satisfactory.

Stevia Should Be Introduced Gradually

Stevia does have negatives. Certainly an initial taste negative. Stevia requires a certain dedication to reprogram your sweetness sensors. The sweet taste of stevia is different from the sweet taste of cane sugar. It took me almost three months before my taste buds completely changed their definition of sweet from cane sugar to stevia. Interestingly, now that most sweetness in my food comes from stevia, foods sweetened with stevia taste "right," but foods sweetened with sugar (or other sweeteners) taste "different." Most commercially prepared sweet foods taste "too sweet." The taste of a commercial donut gags me.

What can you do to help the reprogramming of your sweetness sensors from sugar or high fructose corn syrup (with calories) to stevia (calorie-free)? The best advice I can give you is the one I give for all sorts of positive changes in your eating. Do it gradually.

If one day you give up all sugar-sweetened and HFCS-sweetened foods for only those sweetened with stevia, you will be in for a struggle. (Trust me, on this.) If, however, you gradually begin to replace the sugar-sweetened and HFCS-sweetened foods with stevia-sweetened foods, the transition will go more smoothly. How might this work?

For example, you might reduce the amount of sugar in muffins or a pie you are baking to half what the recipe specifies. When serving the muffin or pie, sprinkle a little of powdered stevia over the muffin or wedge of pie to bring the sweetness level up to normal. Later in your transition to stevia, reduce the sugar amount to one-fourth and compensate with stevia when serving. Gradually you can arrive at the point at which I have been for a number of years: baking without any sugar at all—and adding stevia for the sweetness when serving.

Another example. If you sugar your tea or coffee, you can begin a process using both sugar and stevia. Gradually modify the proportions from mostly sugar to half and half to mostly stevia. Finally, when the taste is "right" for you, discontinue the sugar entirely. Remember that when I advise about proportions here, the proportions are sweetness, not physical amounts. In some types of powdered stevia, 1/16 or 1/8 teaspoon of stevia has the sweetness of one teaspoon of granulated table sugar. More about different types of stevia later in this section.

Too Much Stevia Tastes Bitter

This is the odd thing about stevia. When you put too much table sugar in a food or beverage, it tastes super-sweet. When you put too much stevia in a food or beverage, it tastes bitter. A chemical reason exists for this which I will spare you. Yet I know from years of experience that if I add too much stevia, it will taste bitter.

Many people do not understand how much sweeter stevia is than sugar and have difficulty using a sufficiently small amount to produce a satisfactory level of sweetening. This takes practice, I admit.

These proper amounts of stevia needed to achieve best sweetness vary from brand to brand and in different forms of stevia sold by the same company. Label directions are not a foolproof guide. Usage amounts specified on the label are only a starting point for your own experimentation.

In addition to easy portability, the reason most stevia is sold in little packets that include other ingredients such as maltodextrin is to make it easier for you to use the right amount. If, however, you use the pure powdered form of stevia, getting the right amount sprinkled over a muffin or wedge of pie takes skill. The pure powdered form of stevia is easier to use in beverages. The pure powdered form of stevia I buy recommends 1/64 teaspoon for a serving. Many sets of measuring spoons sold now include a 1/8 teaspoon. Still, it can be tricky getting that 64th measured.

The good news is that for the size cup of coffee or tea most people sweeten, 1/64 teaspoon is not enough. 1/8 or 1/16 teaspoon will probably give the sweetness you desire. Those amounts are easier to measure with a 1/8 teaspoon measuring spoon.

In the early days of my stevia use, I read a post on an online tea discussion group one woman's system for pure powdered stevia to sweeten her cup of hot tea. She had a particular knife that she dipped to a certain point into her hot tea. She then dipped the wet knife point into the stevia powder. The stevia powder that clung to the wet knife point was then mixed into her cup of tea and provided the right amount of sweetness for her. Why did she use the tip of a knife and not the tip of a spoon? Her spoon was too broad to be inserted into the little container of stevia.

Liquid Stevia Works Better For Sweetening Beverages

Liquid forms of stevia have advantages for sweetening beverages, especially cold beverages where there might be difficulty with the powdered stevia dissolving properly.

When I first began using stevia, there were basically two choices in liquid stevias: liquid stevia preparations made with alcohol and liquid stevia preparations made without alcohol. Some stevias in alcohol base are a whopping 20 percent alcohol. (Most wines are only about 11 to 13 percent alcohol.) Though because only a few drops of liquid stevia are used to sweeten a serving of beverage, the effect of the alcohol is negligible.

Liquid stevias without alcohol are often in a water and vegetable glycerine base. I have always found the versions of liquid stevia in the alcohol-free base as acceptable in taste as those in alcohol. But I must include the caveat that I drink very few sweetened beverages so I may not be the best authority on stevia's beverage sweetening.

A survey of available stevia as I was writing this section discovered numerous new varieties of liquid stevia. Some now have various flavorings such as chocolate, vanilla, strawberry. Some claim the ability to sweeten with smaller amounts than previously required.

Do Those Stevia Products Designed For Weight Control Work?

You can find on the market various stevia products that contain ingredients such as inulin and chromium that are claimed to help you use weight by supporting healthy glucose metabolism. My approach to stevia has been to use those types with the fewest additive ingredients. I never bothered to find out precisely what inulin was or was supposed to accomplish. Though I did know that chromium has been shown in testing to help in weight control. More recently I learned that inulin is a non-digestible soluble fiber that can be utilized for nourishment by the probiotic bacteria in your system. Given that recent research that has shown the importance of probiotic bacteria in staying slim, I may be re-evaluating my attitude toward the version of stevia with inulin—and chromium. Though most stevias with these additives advise limited daily use.

Baking With Stevia is Tricky

Baking with stevia is tricky—and not always satisfactory.

I make cakes, pies, cheesecakes, cookies, muffins and jams without sugar, then, sprinkle a little powdered stevia on top before I eat them. That method is so satisfactory for me that I have never done much experimenting with adding stevia to foods before cooking. If, however, you want to experiment with this, you can find any number of stevia cookbooks as well as recipes online.

Stevia Sweetens Some Foods Better than Others

In my experience, stevia seems to work better in foods with higher acidic content. To my taste buds, stevia will do a better job sweetening a slice of my sugarless cheese cake topped with crushed pineapple than it will cinnamon toast in which I have used stevia to replace sugar.

Is Stevia Safe?

Stevia has been touted as a safe sweetener because—unlike artificial sweeteners produced in a laboratory—stevia is natural. (Also because it has been used for centuries in South America without problems.) Stevia, the plant, is actually a member of the daisy family. Doesn't that sound harmless?

But lately, alarmist articles have been appearing in the media about the debate whether or not stevia is truly natural—if the forms that you find for sale have been extracted by a chemical process.

For many stevia products, the extraction process consists of first drying the leaves of *Stevia rebaudiana* and then extracting the rebaudioside by a water extraction process. This is followed by further extraction by ethanol or methanol to isolate the purer form.

Many of us would not have a problem if ethanol is used. That is just another name for drinking alcohol. But methanol is produced in a catalytic industrial process directly from carbon monoxide, carbon dioxide, and hydrogen. What brands use stevia that has been extracted by ethanol and which by methanol? I don't know.

Is the amount of residue left in the stevia that we find in the commercial products enough to worry about? In the past several years, extensive testing has been done on the various kinds and preparations of stevia. No causes for alarm have been reported for moderate daily use. Stevia is so sweet that you use very small amounts. I have found no reason for personal concern so I continue to use stevia—though since, before I switched to stevia, I had already cut back severely on the amount of sugared food I eat, my daily consumption of sweet is low. I sprinkle a little stevia on my breakfast muffin and on the occasional pastry eaten with afternoon tea. Sometimes if the supermarket fruit is particularly blah even when ripe, I will use a little stevia to jazz up the flavor of the fruit.

In the summer, in the blender, I whip up a replacement for ice cream or sorbet with frozen fruit, with or without milk, sweetened with stevia. My favorite summer dessert is stevia-sweetened frozen mango pieces pureed and whipped with cream in the blender. Served in my grandmother's antique sherbet glasses, this desert is delicious to behold—and to taste.

If you are concerned about chemicals used in the extraction process, at least one brand offers stevia powder that is extracted only with water. I tried SweetLeaf Stevia about three years ago. Two negatives: it was more expensive than my regular brand, and I found its sweetening ability anemic.

Doing Your Own Stevia Extraction

You can buy dried stevia leaves and do your own extraction. It is as easy as making a cup of tea—though you may not be terribly pleased with the sweetness you achieve with your extraction.

Recently I ordered organic stevia leaves from Simpson & Vail tea and coffee merchants. Steeping one teaspoon of stevia leaves in 8 ounces of boiling water, did produce a sweet-tasting liquid. But when I followed the instructions to add the one teaspoon of stevia leaves to a teaspoon of an herbal tea blend (I used a blend of rooibos, calendula, rose hips, dried apple and dried orange peel I had been enjoying), the stevia did not sweeten the herbal tea.

Better results were achieved when I steeped one teabag of St. Dalfour black cherry flavored black tea with one teaspoon of dried stevia leaves. The sweetness was subtle, but it was definitely there. And it nicely accentuated the black cherry flavor. Most St. Dalfour black teas are mild Ceylons. I am not sure how sweetening from these home-steeped stevia leaves would stand up in a cup of malty

Assam or some of the hearty breakfast tea blends. For coffee and other beverages, one might steep stevia in high concentration and then add a little of this liquid to the hot coffee or hot chocolate.

You can grow your own stevia. Stevia makes a pretty plant in a pot or in a flower bed. Remember it is in the daisy family, though stevia's white flowers do not look much like a daisy. Nurseries and other outlets sell both seeds and starter plants. Reportedly, the germination rate of stevia seeds is low. To avoid disappointment, you might want acquire a starter plant. I have never grown stevia, but I understand it is much like growing other herbs for cooking and making teas.

Will Stevia Lower Your Blood Pressure?

Are the claims that stevia can reduce high blood pressure true? My answer is yes—and no. Based on my personal experience, I believe that the way stevia can help manage blood pressure depends on what is causing the elevated blood pressure in the individual. For instance, if high consumption of table sugar and high fructose corn syrup has been identified the cause of elevated blood pressure in an individual, then replacing that sugar and HFCS with stevia as a sweetener—other factors being equal—quite likely would bring about a lowering of blood pressure.

But for me, who avoids sugar and HFCS in her diet, I find that whether or not I consume any stevia during the day has no discernible effect on my blood pressure. I monitor my blood pressure daily. The prime regulator on my blood pressure has consistently proved to be exercise. Depending on how much and the quality of my physical exercise during the day, I can usually accurately predict the blood pressure reading on my monitor. If I don't exercise, stevia won't offset that neglect.

Satisfactory Brands Of Stevia

When I first began using stevia, I tried many brands. After a year or two of trials, I settled on the NOW brand of powdered stevia in packets and the company's liquid stevia without alcohol as offering me good quality at a good price.

Then around 2004, we had a spell of humid weather. During that time I found that the thin paper packaging did not protect against the moisture in the air. The stevia powder caked and became unusable. I had to throw out almost an entire box of stevia packets. I switched to NuNaturals' NuStevia whose packaging of powdered stevia offered better moisture protection—and more security against tearing when I put stevia in my handbag or lunch container. I found the quality and price of NuStevia equally acceptable as my previous brand. I have continued to find this stevia satisfactory.

In addition to the packages of powdered stevia, NuNaturals offers stevia powder in a 12-ounce container at an attractive price. Those 12 ounces of stevia provide 672 one-fourth teaspoon servings. I rarely use an entire packet of stevia, so buying stevia in the loose powdered form eliminates the problem of where to keep those little open packages of stevia with their tops folded down that often end up spilling wherever I put them.

For loose powdered stevia I have a small, cut glass dish that holds one and one-half tablespoons of powdered stevia (18 servings) with room for a silver demitasse spoon to use as a stevia scoop. For even more elegant service, I put the stevia in one of my crystal salt cellars.

Summing Up Stevia

Stevia can help you become and stay slim by reducing the amount of calories you consume from sugar and high fructose corn syrup. But it will probably take commitment and some effort on your part to make the transition to stevia—whether you use stevia to provide all, or only a part of the sweetening in your foods and beverages.

New techniques for extracting stevia and new products containing those extracts are constantly being developed. You may have to try several brands and versions of stevia before you find one that suits your taste buds and your budget. From time to time, you may want to try a new stevia product to see if quality has improved. Natural food stores may offer a better selection of stevias than your supermarket. If, like me, you cannot purchase your preferred stevia locally, there are online merchants that sell stevia. For years I have ordered stevia from *iherb.com*.

Without stevia, I could not stay slim—yet still enjoy the quantity and quality of sweet pastries, jams and beverages that I do.

Stevia makes my staying slim sweeter.

Fat is not the problem. If Americans could eliminate sugary beverages, potatoes, white bread, pasta, white rice and sugary snacks, we would wipe out almost all the problems we have with weight and diabetes and other metabolic diseases.

Dr. Walter Willett

Chairman, Department of Nutrition
Harvard School of Public Health

The Réalité Technique

THE REALITY TECHNIQUE

A few years ago, counting calories was the weight control method *du jour*. One bit of humor that made the rounds then was a list usually titled something like "Calories That Don't Count." I do not remember the entire list, but they were things such as the peanut butter you licked off the spoon, the half sandwich left on your toddler's plate, chocolate eaten in the dark.

The humor here (or stupidity, depending on your perspective) was that many Americans following a diet program that required counting calories were not adding into their daily totals calories they kidded themselves "did not really count."

French women would fail to see humor in such a list. They would think that believing that eating certain high calorie foods under certain conditions, such as in the dark, made them calorie-free was idiotic. *Ils sont fous ces Américains!* They're crazy, those Americans.

Yet when it comes to weight control, I continue to be astounded at how many Americans kid themselves about the realities, and how, seeking the easy miracle, they buy the hype. And they buy the gimmicks. $30 billion a year spent on weight control products in the USA. Many of these products are useless. Some are dangerous. Yet despite all the books, tapes, videos, supplements, diet pills, and exercise equipment Americans are getting fatter, and fatter.

Why are Americans less willing than people of other nations to accept the reality of a situation? I think there are historic reasons.

If those who settled this country and turned wilderness into a productive, prosperous nation had focused closely on the realities of the situation, they would likely have stayed in the countries from which they came. If those pioneers in their covered wagons setting out for the western frontier had been realistic about the difficulties and dangers and possible death that lurked in the mountains and deserts, few would ever have ventured out to settle the West. Optimistic avoidance of reality is great for turning harsh, dangerous wilderness into a prosperous, developed nation. But in the 21st century with the geographic frontier tamed, optimistic avoidance of reality about what you are feeding your body can make and keep you fat. It can undermine your health. Avoidance of reality can keep you from having meaningful and successful relationships.

After the attacks on 11 September 2001, many thoughtful people wrote that, in those attacks, Americans had lost their innocence. A better way of stating it was that Americans could no longer go on avoiding certain realities. We had to face the reality that the oceans east and west and the friendly neighbors north and south no longer gave us the protection it once did. We had to stop believing the comfortable myths we had created about our security. We had to face the fact that there were some pretty dangerous people in the world who really, really do not like the USA.

Most of the approximately two-thirds of the population of the USA who are overweight have not yet had a similar wake-up call. They heard the TV anchorwoman read the lead to the story about the US Surgeon General declaring excess weight and obesity a national epidemic and picked up the remote control and switched to the Food Network.

Too many of those who have determined to try to do something to take off excess pounds are buying the weight control books that offer one extreme gimmick or another. Others think charging a StairMaster to their VISA card will do the trick. They somehow neglect the reality that they are actually going to have to work out on the StairMaster on a regular basis to get any results.

So why not face the reality that, instead of extreme programs and expensive equipment, you just need to stop overeating a lot of processed and convenience food and take a brisk walk 30 minutes a day about five days a week? Is that just too simple?

Many women who do face the reality about food and weight control are still unrealistic about men. As I have written repeatedly, French women accept men as they are. Many American women have the idea that they can change men to the way they think men should be. History, psychology, and biology indicate men are not very changeable.

And when men do not change to the way women want them to be, the frustration that results often drives these women to overeating.

One of the people writing the most logically and sensibly about the benefits of being more realistic about people and situations in your life is the psychologist Nathaniel Branden, mentioned earlier in this book. Two of his books deal specifically with this topic: *The Art of Living Consciously* and *Taking Responsibility*.

In *Taking Responsibility*, Dr. Branden has an excellent chapter, "Self-Responsibility and Romantic Love." He discusses how women often avoid the unpleasant facts about the men with whom they are involved, thinking they will be happier that way. But, in fact, these women remain miserable and distraught.

In contrast, he quotes a woman who told him, "An hour after I met the man I married I could have given you a lecture on ways he would be difficult to live with." But she adds, "He's the most exciting man I have ever known. But I've never kidded myself about the fact the he's also one of the most self-absorbed."

She says that she had to realize and accept what she was getting into when she married him, or she would have been upset later. But is she upset? No, she says, "I've never been happier in my whole life than I am right now in this marriage."

She faced the reality of what her marriage was going to be. And nowhere in her statement that Dr. Branden quotes is there the slightest suggestion that she has any thoughts of changing her husband. She looked at the total package and thought that the positives outweighed the negatives.

For an example of a woman who went into marriage avoiding the realities of the situation and experienced great frustration because of it, I can think of few better public examples than Diana, Princess of Wales. As the unhappy saga of the relationship between the Princess and her husband Prince Charles played out in the media, I could not help thinking how much of her anguish might have been avoided—and how much better training for life as the wife of the future king of England it would have provided— if, instead of working as a baby-sitter for an American family in London, she had spent a year or so in Paris working as an *au pair* for a French family. French women would have shown Diana by example how to accept the realities of the men with whom you are involved.

It always seemed to me that perhaps Diana believed the premise in all those romance novels written by her step-grandmother, the author Barbara Cartland. In these novels the "prince" who has had many lovers falls so passionately in love with the beautiful young woman that he marries her and pledges his fidelity for the rest of their days.

Barbara Cartland sold a zillion books and became very rich authoring books built on that romantic premise. But factual historical evidence does not suggest monogamy as a usual practice of British royalty. Had she faced this reality, might not Diana have made a decision that she could or could not live with the realities of marriage to a royal prince and given her answer accordingly? If you listen to that famous interview Princess Diana gave to the BBC, you feel that her fantasy of what marriage to Charles would be like was far stronger than the reality indicated by history and by what anyone could have learned about Prince Charles from the extensive media coverage of the man.

We know from Diana's own public statements that she experienced much mental anguish which led to problems with health and with food as her marital unhappiness grew.

Apparently I am not alone in believing a French attitude toward her marriage might have aided Princess Diana in her dealings with her husband. I received an email from a woman well familiar with the *Chic & Slim* French-inspired philosophy who, after seeing a television film on the royal marriage, wrote:

> While I certainly do not justify some of Prince Charles's actions, I wondered to myself if only Princess Diana had handled him in a French manner, never demanded, never made accusations about Camilla Parker-Bowles, instead charmed him, stayed calm instead of having hysterics etc. that perhaps history would have been very different.

People often confuse facing reality with pessimistic thinking. Facing reality neither sees things pessimistically nor optimistically. Facing reality is simply looking at things as they *are*.

Another reason people avoid reality is they are afraid of the pain that facing reality will bring. They think that it would be better not to know the truth. In fact, avoiding the facts of situations and about people brings the difficulties in most cases. For instance, there are women who insist that their problem with excess weight is hereditary. Often what they "inherited" is their family's habit of eating large servings of dessert at the end of every lunch and dinner and a big bowl of ice cream before going to bed. If they faced the realistic facts about the situation, these women would realize that it was their consumption of more food than their bodies required (much of it nutritionless refined sugar) that was causing their excess weight.

There are women who, as young girls, were told by their mothers, or their cousins, or their next door neighbor that they were unattractive. They continue to believe this as adult women. But if they were realistic about their features, they would realize that there is nothing wrong with their looks. All they need is a better haircut, new eyeglass frames that suit them better (or contact lenses), altering their skirt length to a more flattering one, and trading their comfortable shoes for a stylish well-made pair of mid-heel pumps, some sexy sandals or boots. Probably better posture would also help. In many cases, being told as a child that you are unattractive is a real posture killer in the adult woman.

Now there are an astounding number of safe and reasonably-priced cosmetic procedures that can correct facial and figure flaws. Many of these machines and related treatments were developed in France.

Americans also refuse to face certain realities about food. I knew a woman in the 1960s who insisted that Sprite was a diet soft drink. None of us could convince her that Sprite contained sugar, and if she wanted a non-cola carbonated beverage, she would do better to choose Fresca. She continued to drink Sprite and was only mildly puzzled when, instead of losing weight, she actually gained about 10 pounds. Read the labels of the foods and beverages you eat and drink.

In his book *The Art of Living Consciously*, Nathaniel Branden stresses that people learn to avoid reality because experiences as children forced them to do so in order to survive bad parenting. Yet he says that the benefits of being conscious of the true facts of a situation are well worth the fantasies one gives up. "In aligning ourselves with reality as we understand it, we optimize our chance for success. And in setting ourselves against reality, we condemn ourselves to failure."

The sultry Latin beauty Bianca Jagger said, "It is when you understand yourself, really know who you are emotionally, mentally, and physically, that real beauty emerges."

Knowing yourself requires being realistic. So to achieve real beauty, too, requires being realistic.

You can greatly increase your chance for being slim, healthy, happy, attractive, and successful if you avoid kidding yourself, and if you accept and deal with realities in your own life.

How You Do It For Chic & Slim Success:

✒ Ask yourself in what areas of your life you are avoiding the realities about food, about people, about yourself?

✒ If you are afraid of certain realities, ask yourself what might happen if you were to accept the reality of the situation, what would you do differently than you are doing now? If you approached the situation differently, might the situation improve?

✒ Do not allow people's perceptions of people and situations to determine your own understanding of people and situations. Make your own analysis and make up your own mind about what the reality is. Get facts, not opinions.

✒ Accept the reality that quick weight loss schemes and gimmicks only work in the short term. If you are overweight, in the long term, you are going to have to modify your lifestyle if you are going to lose weight and stay slim and healthy. And take it from someone who modified her lifestyle, the rewards are definitely worth the efforts to change.

Frenchwomen have been in the professions for years—as doctors, lawyers, professors, writers, businesswomen—without threatening their men nor relinquishing one iota of their feminine appeal in exchange for success. At her best, the Frenchwoman is a compendium of worldliness, chic, charm, mystery, and subtlety who realizes that a feminine woman can create an aura of beauty without being beautiful at all and can do whatever she pleases as long as she does it with taste and discretion.

Diane de Dubovay
on Femininity in Vogue

The Féminité Technique

THE FEMININITY TECHNIQUE

Femininity is the quality of being womanly. French women are known for being the *plus femme*, the most feminine women in the world. They have raised femininity to an art form: *l'art de femme*, the art of being women. Their femininity, rather than costing them in the workplace, seems to pay dividends.

Karen Fawcett, president of *bonjourParis.com,* wrote in an article on that website: "In France, it's OK for women to look sexy." But, she explains, "French women don't wear see all/show all clothes to the office. However, don't be surprised if you encounter a female bank executive wearing a dark suit with a short and tightly fitted skirt, a silk blouse showing a bit of décolleté and very high-heeled shoes." Karen Fawcett adds that, with few exceptions, in France, executive women are taken seriously. They don't have the kind of sexual harassment laws in the workplace we have in the USA because French women "are perfectly capable of fending for themselves."

French femininity is neither lacking in intelligence, nor weak and helpless. Quite often these very feminine French women are perfectly capable of hoisting a wrench and unplugging a stopped-up sink, and still looking adorably feminine as they do so.

Certainly what she chooses to wear is an important element in French women's femininity. But even when actively participating in sports, French women usually manage to make themselves look feminine. Recently I was looking at a snapshot of two young

Frenchmen and two young Frenchwomen on an Alpine hiking jaunt. They had stopped to pose for someone's camera. The young women were wearing jeans, hiking boots, a pullover sweater, and caps. I have seen numerous photos of a hiking excursion that included young American men and women. Why did these French women look so much more feminine than the young American women I have often seen in hiking photos?

First of all, these young women were chicly slim (so often American women these days are chunky) and their jeans were worn very tight and rolled just so to just below the knee leaving an expanse of shapely calf between the top of the boot and the pant. Their sweaters clung so that they showed their bust to advantage, and the caps on their heads sat at just the right angle. They looked into the camera so sure of their attractiveness. Ah, that element of French confidence does so much for attractiveness. More than anything they look comfortable in their own skin and pleased with being women.

In *The Parisian Woman's Guide to Style*, Parisian mother and daughter Virginie and Véronique Morana show us those chic feminine clothes that enhance and define French women's femininity. One section "Lingerie: Quintessential Feminine Allure" begins: "Marked by elaborate detail and fine fabrics, good-quality French lingerie tends to be fairly expensive." The authors define the various categories of French lingerie according to price and style. The list begins at the top. "The quintessential name in Parisian lingerie, Christian Dior, is the most luxurious—and most expensive."

An introduction I often use when I give talks to women's groups about *Chic & Slim:* I hold up an aerobic exercise videocassette and say: "American women find this product useful for weight control." Then I hold up a Christian Dior lavender lace underwire bra and say: "While American women find an aerobic exercise videocassette useful for weight control, French women find pretty feminine lingerie useful for weight control." That is the best way I know to briefly explain the different approaches French women and American women have for staying slim.

French women often invest in quality lingerie. They believe it pays rich dividends in how they feel about themselves as women. Even when no one else sees it. Though these women are very good at deft little movements so that some of their lingerie just happens to show. For instance, when they bend down to pick up Fido, a jacket falls open in such a way to give a glimpse of the bodice of a lacy slip.

In the USA today, you can buy feminine, lacy, well-made lingerie for reasonable prices. You can use it as your secret weapon for feeling feminine.

Care of their bodies to keep them soft and pretty is also a strong element in French women's femininity. Diane Johnson, in her Paris-based novel *Le Mariage,* describes the young French woman Anne-Sophie d'Argel:

> Anne-Sophie, at home in her small apartment on the rue Saint-Dominique was preparing to bathe. Rosy and compact, her breasts were the little pink-tipped breasts of a Boucher nymph.... Nipples just peeking out of the suds. . . polished toe surfacing at the faucet end. Anne-Sophie lined up the stuff she used for her elaborate baths: bath oil, soap, shampoo, rinse, *crème de gommage*, razor, pumice.

Diane Johnson tells us that Anne-Sophie believes in paying attention to the *petits soins*, the little personal care details that keep a woman pretty and feminine.

A bit later she writes about Anne-Sophie's attitude toward her upcoming marriage to a young American journalist: "Anne-Sophie had a Frenchwoman's sense of vocation—but she was also an expert in hunting prints and a very good businesswoman." Anne-Sophie had a very strong French sense of her vocation as wife, but that in no way precluded her from having a successful and interesting career.

What aids a woman's femininity? What diminishes it? We already see from some of the above examples that practicing the French brand of femininity certainly does not stop a woman from holding an executive position, nor from running her own business. So. Is femininity basically a few well chosen accessories, valuing oneself enough to take care of one's body with regular grooming, and believing that an appearance and personality pleasing to men is a useful aid to achieving one's own happiness?

I received an email from a woman who had bought and read the *Chic & Slim* books. In her letter, she included the paragraph:

> In addition to helping me lose weight, you have also helped me reconnect with my femininity. Throughout my weight problems, I've still felt attractive, but not especially feminine. Now I'm taking the extra time in the morning to put on some pearl earrings or a sparkly pin. Just an extra touch to give me that "chic" edge.

How does a woman make herself more feminine? In the Irving Berlin musical *Annie Get Your Gun*, the character Frank Butler, based on the real life husband of legendary markswoman and show personality Annie Oakley, defines the traits of a feminine woman in a song, "The Girl That I Marry." As I write this, I am listening to Tony-nominated Broadway star Tom Wopat sing the song on the soundtrack of the 1999 Broadway Revival of *Annie Get Your Gun,* in which Bernadette Peters played the title role. The list of femininity traits from the song seem very much in sync with French femininity.

Beginning the list is the declaration that a feminine woman

is *soft and pink*. That would certainly mean caring for the skin, especially the face, not to mention keeping rough skin on the feet banished with a pumice stone. French women do not neglect their feet. They also keep the whole body smooth with careful exfoliation. It takes such little time and feels so good, not to mention what a positive payoff in smoother, healthier skin.

The song goes on to say that a woman would *wear satins and laces and smell of cologne*. Satins and laces are often the fabrics of choice in the lingerie French women wear to make them feel pretty and feminine. And a French woman feels undressed without her scent. Helene Rochas said perfume was the "music of the heart." Scent lingers longest in the memory.

Her nails will be polished and in her hair *she wears a gardenia*. French women give great care to their hands and to their nails, though if they opt for nail polish, it will most likely be clear or a pale color. They think dark colors of nail polish might chip and look tacky. But they do usually polish the nails on their well-pumiced, pretty toes in a bright color. Red is a classic choice. One way French women add a note of femininity, even when they are wearing very severe styles such as jeans and a man's shirt, is some adornment for their hair: a hair ribbon, a bow, a barrette or clasp, a colorful scarf as a headband, or even a fresh flower.

She'll purr like a kitten. French women know the power of a pleasing, seductive voice to charm a man. And they are careful to keep their laughter soft and ladylike. No guffaws, chortles, or cackles. Those would not be feminine. A sexy little giggle, however, is another matter.

A doll I can carry. Oh dear! In my fatty days, hearing that last feminine trait listed in the song used to depress me. I was definitely too heavy for any man to lift, at least without serious back strain. But, of course, French women keep themselves slim enough to be easily lifted in a man's arms and carried.

Different men find different feminine elements alluring. Some like polished nails. Some want their wives and girl friends to wear long hair even when hair down below their shoulders is not particularly flattering to these women. Flattering doesn't seem to be the point. So it probably makes sense for these women to go ahead and wear the unflattering hairstyle if it makes the men with whom they have a relationship happy.

Sometimes what a particular man will want the woman in his life to wear is just tacky. (Some American men have really awful taste.) For a woman of good taste this poses a dilemma which requires some diplomacy. One would hope that this hazard could be negotiated without having to choose between wearing something tacky or finding another man.

French models of femininity abound. Catherine Deneuve and Anouk Aimee are *ne plus ultra* examples we have been observing for decades. Lately we have been entranced by actress Audrey Tautou, who so delectably portrayed the lead in the film *Amelie: The fabulous destiny of Amelie Poulain.*

But femininity is more than keeping your toes pumiced, your nails buffed, your lingerie silky, your hair ribboned, and cultivating a pleasing voice. Feeling womanly is a state of mind. And French women find it a most pleasurable and effective state of mind. French femininity is a potent force in their battle against fat.

Vive la femme!

How You Do It For Chic & Slim Success:

⤙ If you don't have one, learn a skin care program appropriate to your skin type.

⤙ Like French women, spend more on skin care than on makeup to cover up skin problems.

➤ Like French women, understand that what you eat and whether or not you exercise regularly will make as much difference in your skin as what you rub on it.

➤ Keep your body exfoliated and smooth.

➤ Keep your nails filed and your hands soft with lotion. Especially if you have to have your hands in water a great deal or you handle paper a lot (paper is drying) be sure to have hand lotion handy to apply often to your hands. Bathroom, bedroom, kitchen, desk, vehicle, and handbag.

➤ Run your fingernails over a bar of soap before gardening. The soap keeps the dirt out and washes out easily with water and a nail brush when your gardening is finished.

➤ Buy a pumice stone to keep your feet smooth. Buy the real stone not the fiberglass version.

➤ No matter what else you are wearing, make certain that you have one feminine element in your outfit.

➤ Choose and wear a signature scent. Even some of the less expensive colognes or *eau de toilettes* have lovely fragrances.

➤ Make pretty lingerie your secret weapon to make you feel attractive and pretty.

➤ Tailor your femininity to the man in your life (or the sort of man you would like to have in your life). Observe him watching other women to see what attracts him.

➤ A relaxed, genuine smile that reflects the true contentment you feel with your life is the best thing you can put on your face.

chic & slim Email to Anne

Hello Anne,

I just wanted to thank you for your website and your postings. I read them daily and always find them thought provoking as well as entertaining. These days, reading them provides a pleasant sense of civilization which you so inspire. I also love your sense of humor. Thanks again, Anne.

Cynthia in Naples, Florida

Bonjour Madame Barone,

I have greatly enjoyed both books—the first one I read in several hours the first night I got it ! I have also scoured your website and find it both informative and enjoyable! Thank you for making this available. I have been trying to find a "fit" for myself — somewhere between Birkenstock-wearing simplicity seekers (simplicity, yes, but no Birkies!) and the all out, jumbo-size-it consumer society in which we live. You make it seem easy !

Elizabeth in Atlanta

Dear Anne,

Can't tell you how much continuing help I get from keeping your book at work and reading it as I enjoy lunch. Keeps me focused on higher thoughts, rather than mindless partaking calories. Thanks, as always, for your contribution to the lives of chic n' slim women everywhere!

Karen Noske

The Toujours Technique

THE CHIC & SLIM ALWAYS TECHNIQUE

French women know that a perverse law operates in the universe.

The law states that if only once in one hundred times you do *not* do something, that will be the one time that it was important that you *do* it.

You can go out with your makeup well applied 364 days a year, but the *one* day that you decide that you can dash out for a quick trip to the convenience store without even bothering with lipstick, that will be the day you encounter (a) the man you most want to see you at your best, (b) your worst enemy who will tell all over town how awful you looked, (c) your always impeccably dressed great aunt who will be very disappointed in your appearance and decide to leave her Waterford crystal to your cousin instead of you. On a really bad day, you will encounter all of the above mentioned individuals.

Generally you eat at mealtime and seated. But on the day that you have a five o'clock meeting, you haven't had time for lunch and you are starving. So as you take the elevator to the 22nd floor, you try to eat a tuna sandwich on the way to the meeting. Of course, just as your mouth is really full, the elevator door opens and into the elevator steps the supervisor who will make your next performance evaluation. You can't even say hello through the wad of fish and mayonnaise in your mouth.

Such stress-producing situations never happen to French

women. They always go out neatly dressed, with their hair and makeup perfect. They would never even think of eating while walking. (The poor digestion, how it would suffer! You would not have pleasure in your meal.)

In Dorothy Adelson's book, *Roughing It On the Rue de la Paix,* she describes her French friend Simone as her "model par excellence of the *femme élégante*." She writes of Simone: "Deeply and irretrievably coquette, Simone would have dressed, massaged, beauty-masqued and creamed to the nines if alone on a desert island."

Mais oui. But, of course, says the chic French woman. Because as everyone knows, *ma chère,* ships sometimes pass by desert islands. And on ships you are most likely to find men. And if a ship passed by, the men aboard would not bother to rescue an unattractive woman. Ah, but one they found pleasing to the eye, they would bring her on board and treat her like a queen as they carried her back over the seas to France.

That is how French women think. These women have their own best interests in mind. Consequently a French woman would always take care of her personal appearance even if she were alone on a desert island.

Several years ago I had major surgery. Every morning around 6:00 AM, the doctor came by on his morning rounds. Having been indoctrinated in the Always Principle by French women, I made it a point to put on my makeup and have my hair combed by the time the doctor arrived in my room.

I was still attached to an IV I had to drag into the bathroom with a decent light. I was still very weak at this point and to do my makeup I had to brace myself against the basin. The IV needle in the vein made it difficult to lift my arm to apply makeup.

One morning the doctor arrived ten minutes earlier than usual. Finding the hospital bed empty, he traced me to the bathroom where he found me propped, wired, and stapled, struggling to draw a line with my eyeliner pencil.

"What on earth are you doing?" he demanded.

I thought it was pretty obvious. But I said, "I am putting on my makeup."

"But you are in a hospital. It's six o'clock in the morning!"

"Look," I told the doctor, "I would put on my eyeliner if I were going to my execution."

No French doctor would have questioned why a female hospital patient was applying her makeup before dawn. A French doctor would have understood that a woman who took care with her appearance would exercise that same care whether she were hospitalized, at a fashionable resort, or on her way to her office. Personal care is something you do *always*.

This is why it is so vital that you have a personal style that is manageable under most circumstances. As I have written in both the original *Chic & Slim* and in *Chic & Slim Encore*, French women's golden rule of chic is "keep it simple." If you design a simple and manageable personal style, you can maintain that personal style on a *toujours*—always—basis.

If you are a mother of young children who require a great deal of your time and mental energy, until they are older and able to do more for themselves, it may be necessary to keep your personal style simple.

As for eating moderately and sensibly, the French do this on a consistent basis. If they do partake of one of those multicourse marathon French haute cuisine meals, say at a Michelin three star restaurant, then they are careful to eat lightly for several days before or after. And sometimes both before and after. They always eat moderately and sensibly in each course no matter how many courses are served at the meal. Remember second helpings are considered impolite in France.

I offer you another story about my incorporation of the French Always Principle into my American lifestyle. When you are living among the French, its easier to maintain the practice of eating moderately and sensibly because that is what everyone does. (And I receive email from other women stating that they had no problem eating sensibly in France, but back home in the USA is another matter.)

When I returned to live in the USA, I was attending dinners with family and friends. Especially for holiday dinners when the others were overeating, I was obvious for my restraint. So I decided that on two days each year, Christmas and my birthday, I would allow myself to eat anything and as much as I wanted. The next Christmas, in addition to all the turkey, dressing, cranberry sauce, rolls, and vegetables, I ate three pieces of pie. One with Christmas dinner, one with afternoon tea, and one with supper.

It is impossible to describe to you how miserable with indigestion I became. My body was no longer accustomed to a large quantity of food, particularly such a large quantity of refined sugar that I consumed in those three pieces of pie, one of which was pecan. (I think another was coconut cream.) About 8:00 PM that evening, I thought I would die of pie. Overeating spoiled my Christmas Day.

When my birthday rolled around the next summer, I still ate "anything and as much of it as I wanted." But the amount that I wanted was much more reasonable. I was restrained from overeating by not wanting my birthday spoiled by indigestion and by feeling as miserable as I had on Christmas.

Before we leave the subject of holidays, I want to caution you about overconsumption of alcohol at festive celebrations. My son tells me that, among his generation, even Halloween has become an excuse to drink to excess. Overindulgence in alcohol (at any time) can put a lot of excess sugar calories into your body. Excessive alcohol also weakens your self control. It can destroy all those good intentions to eat moderately and sensibly. I was always impressed at how restrained the French women I knew were in their alcohol consumption. Being intoxicated and silly (and possibly throwing up) is not chic.

If you are making changes in your lifestyle, it will take a while to get your new systems in operation. Do not worry if you are not hitting 100 percent of Always at first. No one is keeping score. This is not the Olympics. This is *your life*. Just do as well as you can, as much of the time as you can.

Gradually your body will become your ally as my body has become my ally. These days if I overeat or if I overindulge in sugar, then I don't have my usual energy level. I find myself avoiding highly sugared items and restricting my quantity of food. I have things to do, and I cannot work efficiently if I am suffering indigestion. I will not have the energy to function efficiently if I overeat or eat the wrong foods.

If I find myself walking and sitting with a slouched posture, or chattering when it would have been more in my self-interest to have listened quietly, or doing anything more typical of my fatty life than my improved *Chic & Slim* lifestyle, I spend some time thinking how I might have better handled that situation. I look for opportunities to put myself in a similar situation to practice a positive handling of that situation. I remind myself that the more I do something, the more proficient at it I will become, and the more automatic that action will become for me.

So it is extremely important when you design your personal style that you choose ways of living, eating, and dressing that are possible within your financial and time limitations. So you can achieve that style *always*.

In author Francesca Stanfill's, "Fashion or Folly: In these trying times, fashion still matters" in the March 2002 *Town & Country*, she reminds us that when a woman *always* takes care of her appearance, it is not out of vanity, but rather self-dignity and courtesy for others.

Francesca Stanfill ends the article telling readers how French designer Coco Chanel believed that a woman should always make herself presentable before she left the house, because "that day she might have a date with destiny. And it's best to be as pretty as possible for destiny." *Toujours.*

How You Do It For Chic & Slim Success:

➤ Whatever defeating habits and practices you have decided to eliminate from your lifestyle, never do them.

➤ Whatever positive, beneficial practices are going to be part of your *Chic & Slim* lifestyle, practice them consistently. Do them *toujours*—always.

Special Bonus Resource

For You Not As Slim As You Wish
For You Who Want To Stay Slim Forever

One staying slim truth I have learned: for various reasons many people *really* do not want to become slim. Not really. They think they do. But blocks—many of which they are totally unaware—always sabotage their best efforts.

Another staying slim truth I have learned: those who have always been effortlessly slim (eat what they want, never overweight) are too often defenseless when they find themselves victim to a stressful life situation that gives the Fat Monster a chance to get them in her clutches.

If you have long struggled to shed excess weight, but are not yet as slim as you wish, this special section is a do-it-yourself workshop designed to help you analyze your own unique reasons why becoming slim is difficult for you.

If you are among the fortunate effortlessly slim, this bonus section will make you aware of weight gain pitfalls and how you can avoid them.

Tip For Using This Resource

Writing answers to questions posed in the following two special sections can greatly increase their effectiveness for you. A small notebook, sticky notes, using space on this page, notes in a word processing program—whatever paper or digital method you prefer—can clarify your thinking.

Life, Love, Advertising?

WHAT'S SABOTAGING SLIM?

"Tell me what you eat, and I will tell you what you are," so goes that famous dictum of French food authority Brillat-Savarin.

If you tell me that you regularly eat bacon, eggs, pecan sticky buns, and four cups of coffee with cream and sugar for breakfast; two doughnuts for a mid-morning snack; pizza for lunch; nibble on candy all afternoon, and eat fried chicken, baked beans, mashed potatoes and gravy, white bread, Jell-O salad with canned fruit cocktail, and banana cake for supper; a large bowl of chocolate ripple ice cream about bedtime, and drink sugared iced tea with your meals and four cans of cola a day, I will tell you that you are fat.

(If you eat that way 365 days a year and are slim and healthy, then write a book and tell the rest of us how you do it.)

If you tell me that you skip breakfast, drink a diet cola mid-morning, eat a salad (with no accompanying bread or crackers) with low-cal dressing for lunch, and one-half cup yogurt and two steamed vegetables for supper, I will tell you that you are slim—but hungry. And surely lacking *joie de vivre*.

A rigid dietary regime is not necessary for losing weight and staying slim. I know from more than 40 years of personal experience that you can eat meats, breads, cheeses, desserts—good foods you love—and still stay slim.

So if you tell me that you can't become and stay slim no matter what diet or weight control program you try, I will tell you that you likely do not have a good understanding of why you are *not* slim.

YOUR OWN UNIQUE SET OF REASONS

If you not as slim as you desire, it is because of your own unique and individual combination of reasons. Certainly, there are broad general reasons why so many today weigh more than is healthy. But if you want to become slim—or stay slim if you are not overweight—you will need to understand *your own personal relationship to food*.

When I began to study chic French women and what made and kept them slim, I began to understand how my own personal experiences with food had contributed to my excess weight and caused my failure with all the diets I had tried. That understanding was the foundation of my weight loss success. That understanding has been the passport that has enabled me to travel through motherhood, divorce, financial difficulties, and now certain age and still stay slim.

Following are questions designed to begin your process of understanding what is sabotaging slim for you. Or if you are not overweight, how you can avoid pitfalls that would endanger your ability to remain slim your entire life.

Were you fat from babyhood?

When many of us were fat children. Once, a fat baby was considered a healthy baby. Unfortunately, some parents decided that the fatter the baby, the healthier the baby. Did your weight problem begin with parents who overfed you in an effort to make you "healthy"?

Did you grow up in a family where everyone overate and everyone was overweight?

If so, your problem with excess weight may not be not genetics, but simply growing up with bad food habits that must be corrected.

As a child were you rewarded with food for good behavior, as a salve for hurt feelings or to pacify you when you were fussy?

Now that you are grown-up, do you reward yourself with food for a business success, as a salve for disappointment or to calm stress?

Do you still feed your body the same food that you ate as a teenager?

Some people cling to teen food habits as a way of feeling young. Unfortunately, eating like a teen as an adult can lead to fat.

Did the diet-lose-regain-diet-lose-regain roller coaster begin when you were a teen?

If so, it may be time to get off the roller coaster and get on a lifestyle with moderation and healthy eating.

Were you slim until after your first child was born?

A friend went from a size 6 to a size 12 from the time her first child was born and his second birthday. And he was adopted. "It's the stress, not the giving birth," she assured me. Raising young children, especially those with health problems, can be stressful. Too often the stress can put on excess weight. Those chic, very slim French women with three and more children prove that having children does not automatically lead to weight gain.

Did you begin to overeat after a major trauma in your life?

"Every time my husband had to have another surgery," I gained another 15 pounds," one woman told me. A worrying vigil at a hospital can leave you with few food choices other than high-calorie snacks from a vending machine or starchy food from the hospital cafeteria. When a family member dies, friends often bring in food—invariably cakes and other high-calorie foods. So easy to establish bad food habits when distracted by worry or grief.

Did you gain weight when surgery, an injury, or duties caring for an ill family member sabotaged your exercise program?

Eliminating regular exercise can put you on a fast track to weight gain. Determination is needed to restart the exercise program as soon as feasible.

Are you convinced that you were destined to be overweight and have no choice in the matter?

When a child has a strong physical resemblance to family member of an earlier generation, they are sometimes told they are the "physical reincarnation" of that family member. If that aunt or grandparent was overweight, the child sometimes believes that they are doomed to excess weight. Probably not unless their eating habits are the "dietary reincarnation" of that family member.

Do you believe that because diets have not worked for you in the past that you are incapable maintaining a healthy weight?

MInd-sets are powerful. But they can be changed.

What emotions cause you to overeat?

Some of us as children were punished if we showed our emotions. We had to eat our tears, angers, and fears and this became habit that we carried into adulthood.

What takes away your appetite?

Remember the first time you fell in love? Your first big pay raise? Who wanted to eat when you were floating on air.

At which meal do you most often overeat?

Oh please, please do not say all of them.

When you need a snack between meals, do you eat something healthy—or something convenient and quick?

Snacking per se is not unhealthy. But your choice of snacks can make a difference in whether you are overweight or stay slim.

How often do you eat food because someone else pressures you to eat it?

Drug pushers are a serious problem. But food pushers, people who pressure you to eat food you do not want or need, are a more serious problem. Many who would never be tempted by pressure to use illegal drugs, routinely give in to eat food they do not want and put themselves at risk for heart disease, diabetes, stroke, joint problems, even cancer.

Do food and beverage advertisements create hunger and thirst that wasn't there before you saw the advertisement?

Self-mastery requires not responding to every suggestion to which you are exposed.

Are the foods you crave associated with happy memories?

For almost every individual there are foods that carry emotions of a memorable time they were eaten. Often these foods are eaten to re-establish the connections and the emotions of that previous meal. A man, a psychologist no less, told me that he did not like cheese in general, but he loved a particular kind of cheese that he had once eaten on a memorable picnic with a woman with whom he was much in love.

Do you eat high-sugar food for energy pickups?

Sugar is a fickle energy booster, letting you down about as quickly as it boosted you up. Protein is a better energy booster. You will get better sustained energy from a few dry roasted nuts or plain yogurt than cookies or candy.

Do you graze the refrigerator when too tired to prepare a meal?

There is grazing—and then there is grazing. Planning can insure that grazing when too tired to prepare a regular meal offers healthy nutritious foods that require nothing more than removing from refrigerator or pantry and sticking in a fork.

Does a family member chiefly show their love with gifts of homebaked pastries?

A woman who showed her love for her daughter with weekly gifts of a dozen fried pies and a dozen homemade doughnuts presented a problem when the daughter joined a weight control program. The daughter explained that she was trying to lose weight and she could no longer eat pastries so high in sugar and fat. But the next week, here came Mama with the pies and doughnuts. And the daughter said, "But Mama! I told you I was trying to lose weight." And her mother said, "I know you did. That's why I brought you just four fried pies and six doughnuts."

If someone asked you what situation, event or condition was most responsible for making you overweight (or likely to cause you to overeat) what would you say it was?

Let your subconscious play with this. Jot down your ideas and then make comparisons before you define the "most responsible."

Do you really believe that you deserve to be slim and attractive?

Don't waste time pondering this. You DO deserve to be slim and attractive. Chic French women and Anne Barone assure you.

IMPORTANT ADVICE

Understanding what factors contribute to your excess weight can jumpstart weight loss. But *only* if you put that understanding to proper use. Some people have an unfortunate tendency to twist information useful for solving problems into excuses for why the problem can never be solved. Avoid temptation to twist understanding why you are not slim into excuses that sabotage your slim.

The next section is designed to give you more useful analysis to assure your slimness.

Really?

DO YOU REALLY WANT TO BE SLIM?

Before you begin a weight control program, ask yourself if you *really* want to be slim.

You think the answer is yes.

But the answer really might be no.

—Maybe that's the problem.

WANTING TO BE SLIM

Fatty, fatty, two by four, can't get through the kitchen door.

When I was in elementary school, the other children would taunt me with this rhyme as I trudged home from school. I would endure the gauntlet of their painful teasing to my house, where, unfortunately, I could all too easily pass through the kitchen door— straight to the cookie jar.

When I was an unhappy, fat child, I had little understanding of the reasons I was fat. But I knew without one trace of doubt that I truly, truly wanted to be slim. And I knew *why* I wanted to be slim.

I wanted to be free of the painful teasing. I wanted to be able to participate in games without a pain in my side every time I ran. I wanted to be rid of the heat rash between my legs where my fat thighs rubbed together. I wanted to wear pretty clothes like the other girls. Someday I wanted to have a boyfriend.

There was not the slightest doubt in my mind that slim was better than fat. And, I was certainly right about that!

After my years living among the chic and slim French—and my weight loss and wardrobe improvement using their techniques—I returned to live in the USA. Soon I was deeply puzzled by how so many million Americans could be putting so much energy and money into weight loss efforts and having such minimal success. They were either never achieving their weight loss goal—or too soon after losing excess weight, they were regaining it. Why?

Soon it became obvious to me what was really going on. Many of those unsuccessful millions who were putting themselves on diets, attending those weekly Weight Watchers sessions, or toting home bags of Jenny Craig foods did not *really* want to be slim. They felt pressured to do something about their weight. But they did not really want to lose weight and become slim. And they had some very good reasons for *not* wanting to be slim. For many, the price of being slim would be too high.

HIGH PRICES OF SLIM

Too often, food is a sanctuary and compensation, fat is an insulator. People who would never abuse illegal drugs or alcohol find in the overconsumption of starchy, highly-sugared, high-fat foods a legal, affordable, and conveniently available opiate for the discomforts of daily life. Becoming slim would mean giving up the drugs of choice.

Many husbands and partners applaud a woman's weight loss (and write me thank you email when the woman has used the *Chic & Slim* system to shed excess weight). But other men feel threatened by any change, or fear that they might be expected to eat more sensibly too. Some are suspicious an affair is the motive behind the weight loss. So they object to the weight loss, or try to sabotage it. In extreme cases, after a woman achieves a new, slim silhouette, some men break off the relationship. Becoming slim might put unbearable stresses, even end, an important and long-enduring relationship.

Sexual harassment is a problem in all areas of life today. Women encounter it in the office, on the street, in the doctor's examining room—even in their churches. Some women feel that fat is the easiest insurance against harassment. Sometimes this is subconscious. One woman told me that she had never before had a problem with excess weight until she began receiving obscene and threatening phone calls. Before she realized it, she had gained a defensive 10 pounds.

Impossible for me to refute totally that excess fat could be protective. When I was living in India, another American woman there in New Delhi was attacked by her deranged gardener. The knife with which he repeatedly stabbed her in the chest might well have killed the average very slender Indian woman. But the American woman's doctor told her that her fat saved her life. Had she been 20 pounds lighter, the knife blade would have entered her heart. But let me say that unless you have an employee likely to go berserk and stab you with a knife with a relatively short blade, fat is probably more hazard than protection.

Another problem: some worry that if they change the eating habits they learned growing up, it will somehow be a repudiation of their family, particularly their mother who set their eating habits with meals she prepared. One man whose obesity is responsible for many of his myriad health problems justifies his continued eating of large quantities of fried meat and potatoes saying, "This is the way my mama cooked. And my mama was a good woman."

But even good women can have bad food habits that damage not only their children's health, but their own health as well—and deprive themselves of many years enjoying their children and grandchildren.

Following are questions to ask yourself to determine if you really want to be slim—or if the price of losing weight would require paying a price higher than you can afford or would choose to pay.

Have family and friends reacted negatively to your past weight loss successes so that you believe staying overweight will keep these relationships running more smoothly?

Does the active sabotage of friends and family make weight loss too much of a struggle?

If you became slim and attractive, would this have a negative effect on your relationship with your husband or partner?

Do *you* want to lose weight, or do you diet because of pressure from your family, your doctor, or our culture's ostracism of the those who are not slim?

Do you feel that you would be unpatriotic if you ate sensibly and with moderation? Not only American women, but women from other nations as well tell me that their friends and family consider them not truly (whatever nationality) if they do not overeat and binge drink.

Do you feel you would be rejecting your family heritage if you followed eating habits different from what you learned as a child?

Does fat get you out of doing things that you don't like to do?

Does fat make you feel safe?

Do you feel that fat is a punishment for something you did previously in your life for which you have not found any other means of atonement?

What bad things do you fear would happen in your life is you were slim and attractive? Are there no other possible ways you might avoid these calamities?

Do the psychological benefits of staying fat outweigh the damage being done to your health by those extra pounds?

Do you believe that you do not have the right to be slim?

ANALYSIS AND DECISION MUST BE YOURS

No one but *you* can make the "right" decision about whether or not you truly want to become slim. Though anyone making that decision would be foolish not to consider the opinions of their physicians and solid medical research about the health consequences of remaining overweight in making their decision. Do you really want to increase your chances of dying of cancer to avoid tacky comments from that awful woman in your office? Do you want to up your chances of type 2 diabetes because your mother gets upset when you won't eat *two* pieces of her sour cream chocolate cake? Whatever the answers, the choice should be yours.

And what do you do if, after all your careful analysis, you come to the decision that you do not *really* want to pay the price of becoming slim—at least not at this particular stage of your life?

Wouldn't it make sense to stop spending money on expensive special "diet foods?" Wouldn't it make sense to stop spending money on weight control programs when in the end, because you do not really want to be slim, you either do not lose much weight, or you regain the weight soon after losing it?

Some medical studies point out the negative effects on the body of "yo-yo dieting," weight loss followed by regaining the lost weight. And, though I have never participated in a weight control program such as Weight Watchers, I don't think it would be much fun to have to weigh in and be the one who did not lose that week. Or worse, who gained. *(Quelle horreur!)*

If you *really* do not want to be slim, instead of buying those don't-taste-very-good diet foods, why not spend the money on good healthy food you enjoy? Why not take the money you were spending on that weight control program or those exercise machines you never use and buy attractive quality clothes that make you look the most attractive possible at whatever weight you are now?

If you really do not want to be slim, why not avoid those feelings of failure when your latest diet or weight control program does not produce permanent weight loss?

As I told you at the beginning of this chapter, I always knew I wanted to be slim. And more than 40 years experience staying slim, I am totally convinced that slim is a thousand—maybe a million—times better than being fat.

MY OWN ANSWERS TO QUESTIONS I POSED TO YOU

Happily, I avoided many hostile reactions to my weight loss because I was moving frequently during the time I was becoming slim. When I arrived at a new place a size smaller, people at the new place did not know this was not the size I had always been. (And I was savvy enough not to tell them.) For some bizarre reason, Americans are more likely to react with hostility to improvements someone makes. They often greet with glee negative changes. If you gain weight, suffer financial setbacks, have a tragedy in your family, people will love you and be supportive. But lose weight, succeed in making a lot of money, and your children all turn out well, a lot of people will be really, really tacky to you.

That's just the way things are.

As for those negative reactions I did experience, they were like water streaming off a duck's oily feathers. Being slim so improved my life and was such an aid to achieving other goals in my life, that I never, never considered regaining my weight to avoid those negative reactions. In any case, I had friends whose reaction was positive and supportive. I ignored the rest.

After I returned to live in the USA, however, there were many efforts on the part of family and acquaintances to sabotage my weight loss. The lengths to which some individuals will go in order to try to fatten up a slim person are absolutely extraordinary. Most memorable was an effort by a woman during the time I was living in a condo on the Texas Gulf Coast when I was writing the early *Chic*

& Slim books. Mid-afternoon I was taking my regular exercise swim when she came down to the pool carrying a dinner plate heaped with roasted meat, mashed potatoes drowned in gravy, buttered rolls, and some starchy vegetable. Corn, I think. She wanted me to get out of the pool immediately and eat the food.

I thought the woman was insane. To compress a lengthy tale, she repeatedly insisted that I get out of the pool and eat, and I repeatedly declined and kept on swimming. Finally, after about 45 minutes, furious she took the food back to her condo. Fortunately I made her angry enough that she never again interrupted my exercise swim with attempts to feed me a heavy meal. But she did continue to show up at my door with dishes of food.

Weight loss sabotage attempts never end. If you want to stay slim, you must learn to deal with them. Being polite rarely brings relief. You must consistently refuse to give in—even if you make the food pusher very angry.

Happily, all the men with whom I have been involved in relationships were supportive of my efforts to stay slim and dress well. But I know this is not the case for everyone. In situations where a man's inability to deal with the new slim version of the woman leads to a break-up, it is vitally important that she not allow any unhappiness over the ending of the relationship to cause her to eat and regain her lost pounds. This is the time to stay slim so she has a better chance at a new relationship with someone who can appreciate her more attractive appearance.

I am old enough to remember a time when overeating and excess weight were frowned on in the USA—and that was not such a long time ago. From the earliest days of this country's founding, among those of strong religious principle, gluttony was a sin. The idea that overeating to the point of obesity is somehow patriotic is just looney. A nation of wheezing, near-immobile, unfit citizenry can hardly defend the country.

Women who were slim when they were children, but who gained weight after they became adult (perhaps after giving birth) and then lost that excess weight and became slim again have an easier time than women who were fat as children and then become slim as adults. This is certainly true for my generation. For one thing, there just aren't as many of us who were fat children who successfully became slim and have stayed slim into certain age.

In any case, mothers of fat children of my generation were not inclined to take responsibility for their children's weight problems—neither the psychological causes, nor those culinary. As far as my mother was concerned, that I was a fat child was the result of genetic chance just as my younger brother was near-sighted. That my obesity had any connection to those large portions of homemade desserts served every meal except breakfast (where there were homemade jams for toast and pancakes on Sunday) was never acknowledged. So when I discovered the French system of losing weight and staying slim, my mother gave the French no credit. My fat was just something I "grew out of."

With all the junk food and processed food on their plates, what many adult people eat today is so different from what they ate as children that changing one's food habits to healthier ones can hardly be considered a rejection of one's family heritage. For that matter, most of our mothers are not eating what *their* mothers put on the family table. So concerns that our mothers will see as rejection improved eating habits that make us slim seems unlikely. Certainly not likely enough to prevent anyone from shedding unhealthy fat.

Few people will tell you that they can't do something because they are too fat. But often they seem so proud of (and find so useful) their disabilities that their excess weight has caused. For example, knee problems are the excuse so many women give for not walking for exercise. What I find baffling is that they developed knee problems because they became obese because they did not eat sensibly and exercise regularly. And walking is surely one of the least expensive and easiest to perform exercises.

I am known as a champion no sayer. If I decide something is not in my best interest, I do not do it. I certainly do not feel any necessity for endangering my health in order to create excuses for not doing things.

When that woman at one of my seminars told me that she had gained weight in response to obscene and threatening phone calls, I was puzzled. Make her feel safer? Really? If you think you may have to outrun or fight off an attacker, don't you want to be as fit as possible? You will hardly be in your best form if you are carrying weight that comes from fat instead of good, lean muscle. Since I became slim, I have always felt safer than when I was fat and not fit.

Though some people in the Bible Belt milieu in which I grew up tried to convince me that I was fat because it was "God's will," I never bought that explanation. Nor did I ever assign other causes for my fat such as punishment for something I might have done in the past, or that being fat was a part of a universal plan for my destiny. From conversations with the doctors to which my parents took me to find a medical solution for my excess weight, I understood that I was fat because I loved good food, particularly pastries, and because wherever I was, good food was always in abundance. For various reasons, I overate.

At age 13, I did have one weight loss success. Though unfortunately within a year I regained the 20 pounds lost. Yet the experience convinced me that if I could ever discover weight loss techniques that allowed me to enjoy good food, I could become slim. I also got a hint of the role comforting my unhappiness with food played in my excess weight.

Less than a decade later, I found those techniques when I discovered how those chic French women eat all that rich food and still stay slim. And how those women see problems that arise in life not as something negative and distressing, but as the means of making life more interesting. A life without problems would be very boring. *N'est pas?*

When I was fat, I never worried that being slim would have negative consequences. I always believed my life would be better slim than fat. And it has been. That does not mean my life has been without problems. But my problems were caused by decisions that turned out in hindsight to be wrong. And, like everyone, unfortunate things have happened to me over which I had no control. Good things in my life that resulted from being slim have enormously outweighed any problems related to being slim.

I readily acknowledge that some women find psychological benefits from weighing more than is healthy. But this kind of thinking was never a trap that kept me fat. As for a right to be slim, if I ever doubted it, French women convinced me that the right to *beauté* rated as highly the right to *liberté, égalité, and fraternité.*

Those are my answers to those questions I posed.

But you are not me.

Your life situation, your generation, your background, your goals, your value system—even your nationality—likely are different from mine. So you may not choose slim at this time. Perhaps the right choice for you now is *Chic & Healthy.*

Whether your choice is *Chic & Healthy*, or, like mine, *Chic & Slim*, the 10 techniques in this book will help you achieve the goals that you define for yourself.

Think of these techniques as a passport that will allow you to travel to all the exciting and pleasure-filled places you want to go.

Bon voyage.

chic & slim Success

THE KEY

So where do you begin?

You may want to try all of these techniques and ideas at once. *Non, non! Pas une bonne idée.* Not a good idea.

Those of you familiar with my *Chic & Slim* philosophy know I believe the key to permanent positive change is a gradual approach. Try to change too many eating and lifestyle habits at once, your mind and body will revolt. (That is one reason traditional 'diets' fail.) A gradual approach will also allow your friends and family to adjust to the "new you." They will be less likely to try to sabotage your success because they are uncomfortable with the new person you have become.

So where should you begin?

Seek out *le plaisir*, the pleasure element. Which technique seems to you that it would be the most fun? Which technique is likely to give you a quick sense of accomplishment? Which technique uses only items that you already have on hand? Start with that technique. Then move on to others that seem fun to you.

If any of the techniques seem unpleasant, boring, or make you uncomfortable, skip them. You are unlikely to be successful forcing yourself to do something you do not enjoy. Didn't you do enough things you did not enjoy back when you were following one "diet" or another?

Some advice: Do not announce that you are following a program aimed at becoming chicer and slimmer. In the first place, that is very un-French. Those chic French women do not talk about living a healthy lifestyle, they just do it. They do not talk about building a chic wardrobe, they just buy or sew the clothes and wear them.

Besides, if you talk about your program, you will only be setting yourself up to be bombarded with negativity by tacky, jealous individuals who want you to fail. Remember, if you tell your coworkers that you are trying to improve your eating habits, as soon as you lose two ounces of the 25 pounds your doctor says you should shed, one of those coworkers will start warning you about the dire consequences of anorexia.

More advice: Skip the competition. Becoming healthier and more attractive is not a sporting event where someone else has defined the rules of the game and where someone has to win and someone else has to lose. *You* determine your *Chic & Slim* goals. *You* make the decision as to when you have achieved those goals.

More advice: Skip the guilt. If you intended to take 20 minutes to eat your dinner slowly and carefully, and you wolfed it down in seven minutes flat, skip the guilt. Try again next time. Learn the French shrug. A shrug is a marvelous alternative to feeling guilty. Shrugs are French. Guilt is not.

The ideas and techniques in this book are suggestions, ideas, possibilities, avenues. Tailor these techniques to suit your own lifestyle and your own needs and preferences. Some years ago there was a perfume advertisement featuring a ravishingly chic French woman and the blurb beside her said: "You know enough to make your own rules."

Make your own rules. Enjoy your own unique *Chic & Slim* success.

Bonne chance! Good luck!

Anne Barone

Merci Beaucoup

Sometimes writing and publishing a book is much like losing weight. You might, as the ads tease, "lose 30 pounds in 30 days," but most likely the lost pounds would not stay off for the long term. Likewise, I might whip out a new *Chic & Slim* book in a month or two. But most likely the book would not prove useful to you in achieving the kind of chic and slim success you desire. And much thought, much evaluation, and much rewriting and redesigning go into a book that effectively communicates French lifestyle and techniques.

So my first and sincere thanks goes to all the *Chic & Slim* readers who so patiently tolerated the long delays and who sent encouraging email and notes when I was growing increasingly frustrated as a steady stream of unforeseen events delayed completing the book.

Looking back more than a decade since I began work on the original *Chic & Slim*, I remember with gratitude so many who have helped my efforts. The initial idea came from my physician Dr. Robert Hillis who kept saying, "You ought to write a book." I did write a book, and now more books. *Chic & Slim* has grown from an idea into my life's mission. I am deeply grateful for Dr. Hillis's initial suggestion.

My son John remains my most loyal support. Without his help and without his understanding for his mother's obsession to publish her *Chic & Slim* message, I could never have persevered. The friendship and help of Sheryl and Bob White, Betty Buchanan and Ann Davis has been invaluable.

Hurston Daniel Morris generously donated a wonderful and extensive collection of clippings and books dealing with French women for the *Chic & Slim* background materials library. The mechanical expertise of Gene Warren of Warren Imports has kept my vehicles in top condition. The crew at the Morningside Station

Post Office provides wonderful service for shipping the orders of *Chic & Slim* books. Cynthia Seymour's marketing efforts have boosted *Chic & Slim* book sales.

For this book, *Chic & Slim Techniques*, Joyce Wells turned her practiced teacher's eye on the many errors in my manuscript pages. I have tried to correct all of them. If you still find errors in the book, those errors are mine, not Joyce's.

My prepublication readers provided invaluable advice (and entertaining comments penned in the margins). Some readers agreed to be recognized. Others preferred to remain anonymous. I thank Virginia Bandremer, Cynthia Seymour, and my son John for taking the time to read every word of *Techniques* and make suggestions for its improvement.

For the updated 2013 version of the book, *merci* to Ruby in London and Ann-Marie in Kansas City whose enthusiasm for *Techniques* prompted me to bring out a refreshed edition.

Just as surely as the French love good crusty baguettes, I am certain the moment I release this book for publication, I will remember others who really, really deserve to be thanked for their help and support. For all of you, named and unnamed in this acknowledgment, you can take satisfaction that your efforts have enabled many to live healthier, happier, more successful lives, and to develop their own personal styles that are unique—and certainly chic.

My sincerest thanks to all of you. *Merci beaucoup!*

be chic

stay slim

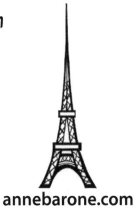